Improving Behavioral Health Care for U.S. Army Personnel

Identifying Predictors of Treatment Outcomes

KIMBERLY A. HEPNER, CAROL P. ROTH, ERIC R. PEDERSEN,
SUJEONG PARK, CLAUDE MESSAN SETODJI

Prepared for the United States Army
Approved for public release; distribution unlimited

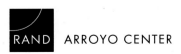

RAND ARROYO CENTER

For more information on this publication, visit www.rand.org/t/RR2829

Library of Congress Cataloging-in-Publication Data is available for this publication.
ISBN: 978-1-9774-0318-6

Published by the RAND Corporation, Santa Monica, Calif.

© Copyright 2020 RAND Corporation

RAND® is a registered trademark.

www.rand.org

Preface

This report documents research and analysis conducted as part of the project entitled *Improving Outcomes Among Soldiers Receiving Behavioral Health Care,* sponsored by the Office of the Surgeon General, U.S. Army. The purpose of the project was to identify key factors that are associated with changes in outcomes and different trajectories of recovery for soldiers who receive Army behavioral health care. This report should be of interest to Army and Defense Health Agency administrators responsible for ensuring excellence in behavioral health care, military providers who deliver behavioral health care to service members, and Military Health System beneficiaries. It should also be useful to those responsible for monitoring the quality of behavioral health care and developing evidence-based strategies to improve behavioral health care for service members.

This research was conducted within RAND Arroyo Center's Personnel, Training, and Health Program. RAND Arroyo Center, part of the RAND Corporation, is a federally funded research and development center (FFRDC) sponsored by the United States Army.

RAND operates under a "Federal-Wide Assurance" (FWA00003425) and complies with the *Code of Federal Regulations for the Protection of Human Subjects Under United States Law* (45 CFR 46), also known as "the Common Rule," as well as with the implementation guidance set forth in U.S. Department of Defense (DoD) Instruction 3216.02. As applicable, this compliance includes reviews and approvals by RAND's Institutional Review Board (the Human Subjects Protection Committee) and by the U.S. Army. The views of sources utilized in this study are solely their own and do not represent the official policy or position of DoD or the U.S. government.

Contents

Figures and Tables

Figures

Tables

Summary

To achieve the goal of psychological readiness for every soldier, the U.S. Army aims to provide the highest-quality behavioral health (BH) care possible. In 2009, the Army recognized a need to centralize BH care to improve coordination and standardization across the service. A key change was integrating BH providers into primary care settings, where they provide support to soldiers with BH conditions through expert consultations, clinical assessments, triage, and brief cognitive behavioral interventions (Hoge et al., 2015). This change has improved access and continuity of care, as well as enhanced communication among primary care providers, BH providers, and unit leaders (Hoge et al., 2015).

To support these efforts, the Office of the Surgeon General, U.S. Army, asked RAND Arroyo Center to identify factors that are associated with changes in outcomes for soldiers who receive Army BH specialty care and to develop recommendations to improve BH care and soldier outcomes.

We identified soldiers diagnosed with posttraumatic stress disorder (PTSD), depression, or anxiety who received BH specialty care and whose outcomes—PTSD, depression, or anxiety symptoms—were assessed during their care. Using treatment data on both outpatient and inpatient care delivered by the Military Health System (MHS) and symptom data collected through an online system that allows for collection of multiple patient and clinician-reported measures, called the Behavioral Health Data Portal (BHDP), we conducted analyses to identify predictors of changes in symptoms (including patient and treatment characteristics) and patterns in symptom trajectories.

Study Methods

Sample Selection

We identified three samples of active-component soldiers who received specialty BH care for PTSD, depression, or anxiety from the MHS between January and September 2016. We allowed a nine-month time frame for sample entry for a new treatment episode—defined as no specialty BH care associated with the diagnosis in the prior six months. We limited our samples to soldiers with a minimal level of symptom severity as measured by the PTSD Checklist for DSM-5 (PCL-5), the nine-item Patient Health Questionnaire (PHQ-9), or the seven-item Generalized Anxiety Disorder scale (GAD-7) (which measure PTSD, depression, and anxiety symptoms, respectively) and those with a second symptom score one to six months after the initial score. Soldiers who may have later separated or deployed but were otherwise eligible by our study criteria were included in the samples. This sample selection followed the approach that the Army uses for its symptom-based outcome monitoring.

Using the sample selection criteria, we identified 3,264 soldiers for the PTSD sample, 3,801 for the depression sample, and 4,282 for the anxiety disorder sample. The three samples were not selected to be mutually exclusive, so it was possible for a soldier to be in multiple samples. The selection criteria likely restrict generalizability, and samples may not be representative of all service members with PTSD, depression, or anxiety.

Data Sources

We focused on administrative treatment data on care provided to active-duty soldiers between December 1, 2015, and June 30, 2017. These files included records on all inpatient and outpatient health care provided by the MHS, including care provided in military treatment facilities (MTFs; direct care) and care provided by civilian providers and paid for by TRICARE (purchased care).

Our analyses relied on symptom score data from three self-report measures, collected using BHDP: the PCL-5 for PTSD, the PHQ-9 for depression, and the GAD-7 for anxiety. These tools are used to document patient symptoms, response to treatment, and remission for patients with initial scores above a defined threshold. We linked each PCL-5, PHQ-9, and GAD-7 score to the administrative data records for soldiers in our diagnostic samples.

We also consulted the literature to identify variables that could affect treatment outcomes. We identified patient and treatment characteristics that have predicted behavioral health treatment outcomes in patients with PTSD, depression, or anxiety and were available in administrative or BHDP data. We grouped these predictors into two categories: pretreatment variables (e.g., demographic characteristics, military service characteristics, comorbid diagnoses and symptoms, and use of health care before the initial elevated score) and treatment variables (e.g., psychotherapy, individual therapy, group therapy, provider characteristics, evaluation and management visits, and medications). Using this process, we defined a total of 57 pretreatment variables and 84 treatment variables, including three covariates that looked at the timing of the initial score relative to the intake visit.

Analyses

Our study consisted of three primary analyses. In the first, we sought to identify patterns in measure completions in BHDP, including how and when measures specific to PTSD, depression, and anxiety symptoms were completed, as well as the amount of time between a soldier's initial score and final follow-up score, the frequency with which soldiers completed outcome measures, and the relationship between the number of BH specialty visits that soldiers received and the number of scores completed. This analysis allowed us to describe the relationship between the number of completed symptom measures and the number of BH specialty visits in the six months after the initial score. We also examined the Army's use of BHDP data to compute and monitor rates of response and remission for the three target conditions.

The second analysis explored the representativeness of our selected samples. These analyses compared characteristics and health care utilization of soldiers in our multivariate analysis samples with a group of soldiers who received at least one direct care BH specialty visit for a target diagnosis but who were excluded for not meeting other eligibility criteria (e.g., soldiers who were not starting a new episode of treatment, whose symptoms were not severe enough at the initial score, or who did not have a second score in one to six months). We evaluated how each study sample differed from the broader one-visit group in terms of demographic characteristics (gender, age, and race/ethnicity), service characteristics (pay grade and deployment history), and health care utilization characteristics (outpatient visits and the rate of co-occurring conditions). We performed chi-square tests (for categorical variables) and t-tests (for continuous variables) to examine whether these variables differed significantly between each sample and our control group.

Our third analysis consisted of two parts. We first sought to identify predictors of outcome for soldiers with PTSD, depression, and anxiety—defined as change in outcome score from the initial score to the last observed outcome score (i.e., last score minus initial score). Developing these models involved a nine-step analytical process that allowed us to identify predictors of PTSD, depression, and anxiety symptom score change. Then, we conducted exploratory analyses to characterize different trajectories of improvement in scores for soldiers who received BH specialty care.

The analyses presented in this report have several strengths, drawing on a range of data sources and identifying variables that had the greatest impact on soldiers' treatment outcomes within and across treatment episodes for the three conditions in our sample. However, the analyses also have several limitations.

The sample studied was limited to soldiers receiving BH care with a new treatment episode, a minimal level of symptom severity, and at least one follow-up symptom score in one to six months. Our results do not include those who received Army BH care but did not have any symptom scores, had less than two scores, or had a lower level of symptom severity at the first visit. Therefore, our results may not generalize to these other populations. Although we examined a lengthy list of variables, we could not analyze all possible variables because they were not included in the available data (e.g., lifetime history of trauma). Furthermore, some variables that we examined may not adequately capture the treatment delivered. For example, we examined a provider-entered variable indicating treatment with evidence-based psychotherapy, but it was not associated with outcomes—a surprising result, given the research support for these therapies in reducing symptoms. The observational nature of the data limited our ability to draw causal links between the predictors and outcomes. In addition, even with the careful variable selection, there is always the possibility of remaining collinearity—highly related variables that could produce biased estimates of the association between outcome and some predictors. With the time difference between the initial and last score varying across soldiers, there is also the possibility of such a time variable moderating (or interacting with) the association between predictors and outcomes.

Findings

BHDP Is Widely Used to Track PTSD, Depression, and Anxiety Symptoms, but There Are Opportunities to Expand Symptom Tracking

Soldiers in all three samples received more scores the longer they were in treatment, suggesting that BHDP has been widely implemented and that soldiers routinely received scores during BH visits. However, we identified areas for improvement. For example, some soldiers had BH visits after their last symptom measure score. Thus, a soldier's last score was not necessarily a measure of symptoms at their last visit. In addition, soldiers in the anxiety sample were less likely than soldiers in the PTSD and depression samples to receive multiple scores; this pattern was more apparent for soldiers with 16 or more BH visits. The Army's monitoring of anxiety symptoms was implemented after monitoring for PTSD and depression, so these results could reflect differing stages of implementation. Further, we identified several differences between the Army methodology for computing depression response and remission measures and similar measures endorsed by the National Quality Forum; these differences make comparisons between Army and civilian care difficult.

Stronger Patient-Reported Therapeutic Alliance Was Associated with Improved PTSD, Depression, and Anxiety Outcomes

Despite using methods to identify the "best-in-class" pretreatment and treatment factors predicting clinical outcomes, we found that no pretreatment variables were consistently associated with outcomes. That is, no demographic or risk factors consistently were associated with all three targeted outcomes within a diagnosis (i.e., change scores, response to treatment, and remission) or across diagnoses. However, one treatment factor was consistently associated with outcomes both within and between diagnoses:

therapeutic alliance. Even when controlling for other treatment factors, a perceived strong working relationship between soldiers and their providers was associated with decreased PTSD, depression, and anxiety symptoms; PTSD and depression response to treatment; and PTSD, depression, and anxiety remission.

Increased Supply of Benzodiazepines Was Associated with Worse PTSD, Depression, and Anxiety Outcomes

Besides therapeutic alliance, no other treatment factor was consistently associated with improved outcomes over time within or across diagnoses. However, a larger supply of benzodiazepines dispensed was associated with poorer PTSD, depression, and anxiety outcomes compared with no supply of benzodiazepines. Although our study did not assess whether soldiers who received these medications used them as prescribed, soldiers with more than a 30-day supply of the drug experienced poorer outcomes.

Many Soldiers' Trajectories of Symptom Change Did Not Demonstrate Improvement

Outcome quality measures currently tracked by the Army—response to treatment and remission based on last symptom scores—showed improvement in some soldiers but also highlighted a need to continue improving the effectiveness of Army BH care. Specifically, rates of achieving either response or remission within one to six months were 35 percent for PTSD, 45 percent for depression, and 41 percent for anxiety. It remains possible that soldiers continued to improve after their last score because our data only captured scores up to six months after their initial score. While one to six months is a relatively short time to evaluate symptom improvement and/or remission of symptoms, some patients have been shown to reach remission of depression within six months (Angstman, Rohrer, and Rasmussen, 2012). Our analyses also identified three or four different patterns, or trajectories, of symptom change for each sample. The majority of soldiers with PTSD (83 percent) were included in a trajectory that did not demonstrate improvement in their symptoms. Among patients with depression, 34 percent were included in a trajectory that showed no improvement, and 45 percent showed a small improvement. Forty-five percent of the anxiety sample were in a trajectory that showed no improvement. Exploring predictors of the trajectories yielded mixed results. Often, predictors that captured increased utilization were associated with a lack of improvement, but it is likely that soldiers who were not improving were more likely to receive additional care. Although we adjusted our models for severity at initial score, there may have been unmeasured confounders that led to these findings.

Recommendations and Policy Implications

Recommendation 1. Provide Feedback on Therapeutic Alliance and Guidance to Providers on How to Strengthen Alliance with Their Patients

A perceived strong working relationship between soldiers and their providers was associated with better outcomes in all three samples, and this finding is consistent with the literature on this topic. Providing clinicians, clinical leads, and MTFs with information about how soldiers perceive their alliance with providers may help providers address difficulties in the therapeutic relationship directly with the patient and use this information as an opportunity to repair the relationship or address concerns about treatment that the patient may have. Provider training in this area may help minimize treatment dropout and improve outcomes. Our analyses were somewhat limited by relying on the last therapeutic alliance score, which was frequently assessed at the same time as the last symptom score, potentially biasing results by increasing the association between these two variables. Therefore, we recommend that the Army ensure that therapeutic alliance is routinely assessed early in treatment. This will ensure that the results of the measure are actionable during treatment for the clinician and that these analyses can be replicated using alliance scores that are collected prior to the last symptom outcome score.

Recommendation 2. Expand Tracking and Feedback on Benzodiazepine Prescribing

One of the most consistent findings in our analyses was that soldiers who had a larger supply of benzodiazepines—more than 30 days—were more likely to have worse outcomes. The clinical practice guideline for PTSD cautions against using benzodiazepines as monotherapy or augmentation therapy for the treatment of PTSD (VA and DoD, 2017), and these medications have been identified as potentially harmful in this population. In 2018, the Defense Health Agency initiated a program to track benzodiazepine prescribing among providers who treat PTSD and acute stress disorder called the PTS Provider Prescribing Profile (Military Health System Communications Office, 2018). Results are monitored and shared with MTF commanders. The Army's Behavioral Health Service Line is also tracking benzodiazepines and atypical antipsychotic prescriptions for PTSD (Woolaway-Bickel, 2019). Data on benzodiazepine prescribing could also be provided to clinic leadership and individual providers as a potential approach to improve patient outcomes, including response to treatment and remission metrics. Additional work could be conducted to identify the duration of benzodiazepine use that may lead to worse outcomes, but our analyses suggest that more than a 30-day supply is associated with worse outcomes.

Recommendation 3. Increase Provider Use of Measurement-Based BH Care

The Army continues to expand and monitor the use of BHDP for BH care. Our sample was limited by our selection criteria, making it difficult to assess the extent of measurement-based care. However, a 2016 survey of BH providers suggested that 76 percent of Army BH providers screened soldiers for PTSD or depression using a validated measure, but only 59 percent reported using symptom data to inform treatment (Hepner, Farris, et al., 2017). Measurement-based care involves the repeated collection of outcome data and the use of those data to inform decisions throughout the course of treatment (Fortney et al., 2016). These data provide timely feedback to providers about patient progress, allowing providers to quickly identify patients who are not improving or deteriorating (Boswell et al., 2015). As the Army continues to expand the use of BHDP and the collection of symptom measures, an important strategy for improving BH treatment outcomes may include supporting providers in frequently collecting and using these data in treatment decisions.

Directions for Future Research

The analyses presented in this report provide results that can guide the Army in improving outcomes for soldiers who receive BH care. These analyses also raised several questions that could be addressed in future research. These include

- *Identifying quality of care measures that can help providers focus on aspects of treatment that have the highest likelihood of improving soldier outcomes (sometimes referred to as "driver" metrics).* These analyses would target therapeutic alliance and supply of benzodiazepines to identify detailed specifications for tracking metrics to assess these variables that are associated with treatment outcomes.
- *Evaluating whether refinements in the definitions of response to treatment and remission currently used by the Army could improve assessment of significant symptom improvement and increases in psychosocial functioning.* Our analyses highlighted that several soldiers who receive at least some Army BH care are excluded from the outcome measures. Expanding inclusion, or developing alternative metrics, may provide more opportunities to more thoroughly monitor the effectiveness of Army BH care. Further, modifications to measure specifications could also improve the ability to compare Army performance with civilian care settings.
- *Exploring the utility of alternative approaches to monitoring Army outcome measures (i.e., response to treatment and remission).* This could include tracking these metrics stratified by populations of interest (e.g., broken out by demographic characteristics or those on a medical evaluation board). Stratified reporting of outcome measures has been suggested as an alternative to complex case-mix adjustment models.
- *Exploring the utility of expanding Army BH outcome monitoring beyond symptom measures.* The Army is a leader in monitoring outcomes of BH care. Thus far, this monitoring has focused on symptom measures. This is a logical focus

because symptoms are the most proximal outcome of BH care and are likely to be improved by high-quality care. However, the Army could explore monitoring other outcomes of BH care. Potential targets could include indicators of readiness, functioning, or quality of life.

- *Developing and evaluating more effective treatments for PTSD, depression, and anxiety disorders.* Our analyses add to existing recent literature that has called for more effective treatments, particularly for service members with PTSD. The observed rates of response to treatment and remission highlight the continued need for more effective treatments within both Army and non-Army settings.

Acknowledgments

We gratefully acknowledge the support of our project sponsors, LTC Deborah Engerran and Kelly Woolaway-Bickel in the Office of the Surgeon General, U.S. Army. We appreciate the valuable insights we received from Lisa Jaycox and Susan Paddock of RAND and Maria Steenkamp of New York University. We addressed their constructive critiques as part of RAND's rigorous quality assurance process to improve the quality of this report. At RAND, we also thank Tiffany Hruby for her assistance in preparation of this report, Dionne Barnes-Proby for her work to oversee human subjects and regulatory protocols and approvals for the project, Emily Butcher for contributing to the literature search, and Elizabeth M. Sloss for her contributions to sections of this report. Finally, we thank Charles Engel and Harold Alan Pincus for their contributions to the development of the analysis plan.

Abbreviations

ANOVA	analysis of variance
AUDIT-C	Alcohol Use Disorders Identification Test–Concise
BASIS	Behavior and Symptom Identification Scale
BF	Medical Expense and Performance Reporting System code for behavioral health clinic
BH	behavioral health
BHDP	Behavioral Health Data Portal
CAPER	Comprehensive Ambulatory Professional Encounter Record
CBT	cognitive-behavioral therapy
CI	confidence interval
C-SSRS	Columbia Suicide Severity Rating Scale
DoD	U.S. Department of Defense
DSM-5	*Diagnostic and Statistical Manual of Mental Disorders*, 5th edition
DSM-IV	*Diagnostic and Statistical Manual of Mental Disorders*, 4th edition
E&M	evaluation and management
FY	fiscal year
GAD-7	seven-item Generalized Anxiety Disorder scale
HEDIS	Healthcare Effectiveness Data and Information Set
ICD-10	International Classification of Diseases, Tenth Revision
ICD-10-CM	International Classification of Diseases, Tenth Revision, Clinical Modification

IOP	intensive outpatient program
LCA	latent class analysis
MDD	major depressive disorder
MEPRS	Medical Expense and Performance Reporting System
MH	mental health
MHS	Military Health System
MN	Minnesota
MTF	military treatment facility
NQF	National Quality Forum
NTE	new treatment episode
OF	occupational function
PCL-5	PTSD Checklist for DSM-5
PDTS	Pharmacy Data Transaction Service
PHQ-9	nine-item Patient Health Questionnaire
PSF	personal/social function
PTSD	posttraumatic stress disorder
SD	standard deviation
SIDR	Standard Inpatient Data Record
SNRI	serotonin-norepinephrine reuptake inhibitor
SSRI	selective serotonin reuptake inhibitor
TBI	traumatic brain injury
TCON	telephone conference
TED-I	TRICARE Encounter Data–Institutional
TED-NI	TRICARE Encounter Data–Noninstitutional
VA	U.S. Department of Veterans Affairs
VM6	Virtual Storage Access Memory Military Health System Data Repository 2006
WRAIR	Walter Reed Army Institute of Research

CHAPTER ONE

Introduction

Overview

The U.S. Army has made a significant effort to improve the quality of behavioral health (BH) care and outcomes for soldiers over the past decade (Hoge et al., 2015). To support these initiatives, the Office of the Surgeon General, U.S. Army, asked RAND Arroyo Center to identify factors that predict changes in outcomes for soldiers who receive Army BH specialty care and to develop recommendations to improve BH care and soldier outcomes. We identified active-duty soldiers diagnosed with a new episode of posttraumatic stress disorder (PTSD), depression, or anxiety who received BH specialty care between January and September 2016 and whose outcomes—PTSD, depression, or anxiety symptoms—were assessed during their subsequent care. Members of the National Guard and Reserve, retirees, and family members were not included in these analyses because these populations may be more likely to receive care outside of the Military Health System (MHS), which would not be captured in our analyses. Using treatment data documenting both inpatient and outpatient care delivered by the MHS and symptom data collected through an online system, the Behavioral Health Data Portal (BHDP), that allows for collection of multiple patient and clinician-reported measures, we conducted analyses to identify predictors of changes in symptoms (e.g., risk and demographic characteristics, treatment characteristics) and different symptom trajectories. We used these analyses to inform a set of recommendations to improve Army BH care.

In this chapter, we first provide the background and rationale for the study, including rates of PTSD, depression, and anxiety disorders among service members and specifically among Army personnel; the Army's steps toward innovation in BH care; and how the Army monitors the symptoms of soldiers who receive BH care.

Background and Rationale

PTSD, Depression, and Anxiety Among Soldiers

Among all active-duty service members, 20 percent of service members received a BH diagnosis in the MHS (among 15 BH diagnoses) in 2016, and during the years 2005 to 2016, Army active-duty service members had the highest proportion diagnosed each year when compared with other services (U.S. Department of Defense [DoD], 2017). The percentage of active-duty soldiers with a diagnosis of PTSD (on at least one encounter) increased from around 1 percent in fiscal year (FY) 2005 to more than 4 percent in FYs 2012–2016 (DoD, 2017). Active-duty soldiers had higher rates of PTSD than other active-duty service members in the 2005–2016 period. The percentage with a PTSD diagnosis was higher among service members who had previously deployed, ranging from 0.7 percent to 8.0 percent in this subgroup from 2004 to 2012. Much work has examined common predictors of PTSD in the military population, with increased risk for developing PTSD based on a number of pre-trauma demographic factors (e.g., female gender, ethnic minority status, prior trauma exposure, history of mental health problems), combat severity and nature of the trauma (e.g., combat versus military sexual assault), and lack of post-deployment support from family, friends, and the broader community (VA and DoD, 2017; Xue et al., 2015).

The percentage of active-duty soldiers with a diagnosis of depressive disorder from the MHS increased from under 4 percent in FY 2005 to 7 percent in FY 2015 (DoD, 2017). Active-duty soldiers had higher rates of depressive disorders than active-duty members from other services in FYs 2005–2016. A 2012 meta-analysis of 25 studies estimated the prevalence of major depression as 12.0 percent among currently deployed military personnel, 13.1 percent among previously deployed military personnel, and 5.7 percent among military personnel who had never deployed (Gadermann et al., 2012). Data used in the 25 studies were collected between 1995 and 2010 and found higher prevalence among personnel in the Army (odds ratio of 2.0 [range of 1.6–2.1]), Navy (1.7 [1.3–1.8]), and Marine Corps (2.0 [1.4–2.3]) than among Air Force personnel (Gadermann et al., 2012). Common predictors cited in the research literature of depression among military samples are demographic factors such as female gender and younger age, family history of depression or other mental health disorders, and current co-occurring mental health problems (e.g., co-occurring PTSD and anxiety) (Gadermann et al., 2012; Seal et al., 2009; Sullivan, Neale, and Kendler, 2000; VA and DoD, 2016).

The percentage of active-duty soldiers with a diagnosis of anxiety from the MHS increased from 2 percent in FY 2005 to more than 7 percent in FY 2015 (DoD, 2017). As with PTSD and depressive disorders, active-duty soldiers had higher rates of anxiety disorders than the other active-duty service members during the 2005–2016 period. Risk factors identified in the research literature for anxiety disorders among military samples are similar to those for PTSD and depression, including female gender, deployment history—more specifically, combat severity—and co-occurring mental health disorders (Erickson et al., 2015; Milanak et al., 2013; Pietrzak et al., 2012).

Efforts to treat soldiers with diagnosed PTSD, depression, and/or anxiety have been informed by decades of research with civilian, active-duty military, and veteran samples. For PTSD, there is strong evidence that psychological interventions—mainly those involving trauma-focused cognitive-behavioral therapy (CBT)—can be effective at reducing PTSD symptoms, while pharmacological interventions are promising but still lacking strong evidence to support use of medication alone or use of medication in conjunction with CBT (Institute of Medicine, 2014; Steenkamp et al., 2015; VA and DoD, 2017). For depression, both CBT and pharmacological treatments, either alone or used in conjunction, have a large evidence base for effectiveness (American Psychiatric Association, 2015; Gartlehner et al., 2017; VA and DoD, 2016). For anxiety, the evidence is also promising for the effectiveness of CBT and certain pharmacological interventions, either alone or in combination, to treat a variety of anxiety disorders, ranging from generalized anxiety disorders to panic disorder and specific phobias (American Psychiatric Association, 2009; Bandelow, Michaelis, and Wedekind, 2017; Hofmann et al., 2012). However, with all three of these disorders, evidence varies based on several factors, such as severity of symptoms, treatment engagement, and population targeted in the studies; and most of the randomized controlled studies of both psychological and pharmacological treatments have been conducted outside of military populations with civilians. This is most noticeable for the treatment of anxiety. This makes it important to continue conducting rigorous treatment trials with active-duty military to identify the most effective types of PTSD, depression, and anxiety treatments for this population.

Army Innovation in Behavioral Health Care

To achieve the goal of psychological readiness for every soldier, the Army aims to provide its personnel with the highest-quality BH care possible (Hoge et al., 2015). Like previous conflicts, the wars in Iraq and Afghanistan have stimulated research to understand the effects of war on soldiers' mental health and to improve the care provided to those who are affected (Hoge et al., 2015). In 2009, the Army recognized a need to centralize BH care to improve coordination and standardization. A key structural change involved integrating BH providers into primary care settings. In Army primary care clinics, licensed BH providers provide support to soldiers through expert consultations, clinical assessments, triage, and brief cognitive behavioral interventions (Hoge et al., 2015). This change improved access and continuity of care and also enhanced communication among primary care providers, BH providers, and unit leaders (Hoge et al., 2015).

Also in 2009, the Army introduced the Comprehensive Soldier Fitness Program, which trains soldiers in essential resilience skills to mitigate the psychological effects of exposure to trauma (Cornum, Matthews, and Seligman, 2009). The following year, the

Army implemented an innovative approach to how it staffed BH providers. Instead of maintaining the traditional structure, dividing the workforce into departments based on discipline (e.g., psychology, social work), the Army reorganized BH care into 12 structured programs with an integrated mix of BH personnel from a variety of disciplinary backgrounds, including psychology, psychiatry, psychiatric nursing, and social work (Hoge et al., 2015). The purpose of these changes was to drive more sustainable, cost-effective, and standardized care.

A recent study described the workforce of BH providers across the service branches, including psychiatrists, psychiatric nurse practitioners, psychologists, and master's-level counselors (Hepner, Farris, et al., 2017). It found that the Army BH workforce was almost three times larger than that of the Air Force or Navy, with 2,365 providers, compared with 830 and 892 in the Air Force and Navy, respectively, reflecting the size of the Army relative to the other services (Hepner, Farris, et al., 2017). Relative to other service branches, the Army's BH provider workforce had the highest proportion of master's-level clinicians (56 percent of BH providers). Fewer were doctoral-level psychologists (27 percent), psychiatrists (14 percent), or psychiatric nurse practitioners (4 percent) (Hepner, Farris, et al., 2017). While differences in the BH workforce were identified across service branches, the optimal mix is unknown.

Army Monitors Symptoms of Soldiers Receiving Behavioral Health Care

To help improve BH treatment outcomes, the Army has significantly expanded efforts to systematically monitor treatment outcomes for soldiers receiving BH care. In 2012, the Army deployed the web-based BHDP across its BH clinics. BHDP, developed by Army Medical Command's Behavioral Health Division, is separate from AHLTA, the DoD electronic health record management system (Army Medicine Public Affairs, 2013), and it performs functions beyond AHLTA's capabilities. The Army's intent in implementing BHDP was (1) to improve BH care and the tracking of soldiers' risk through standardized data collection methods and real-time provider viewing capability, (2) to support the use of clinical outcome data in routine BH clinical care, and (3) to use aggregate outcome data to inform meaningful program evaluation efforts to guide the evolution of the Army's BH system of care (DoD, 2016).

BHDP allows BH providers to assess symptoms using standardized measures over the course of treatment and to use these real-time data to monitor clinical progress and treatment effectiveness. Use of outcome data to monitor individual soldier progress and inform adjustments in treatment are core elements of measurement-based care, an approach to service delivery that has been shown to improve clinical outcomes. Measurement-based care has been found to significantly improve patient outcomes when used systematically (Fortney et al., 2016). The Army regularly administers symptom rating scales to BH patients and uses the symptom scores to make patient-level clinical decisions. The most commonly administered measures are the PTSD

Checklist for DSM-5 (PCL-5),[1] the nine-item Patient Health Questionnaire (PHQ-9), and the seven-item Generalized Anxiety Disorder scale (GAD-7), which assess symptoms of PTSD, depression, and anxiety, respectively. These measures are among a core set recommended for routine monitoring of these conditions because they are practical to administer, are interpretable, and have been shown to be reliable and sensitive to changes in the frequency and severity of psychiatric symptoms and functional impairment over time (International Consortium for Health Outcomes Measurement [ICHOM], 2015; The Kennedy Forum, 2015; Weathers et al., 2013). The PHQ-9 is also the basis of a measure endorsed by the National Quality Forum (NQF) to monitor depression outcomes over six and 12 months (NQF, 2018).

The measure responses are scored immediately and are available on a BHDP portal that providers can access from their own computers. Scores and graphs are displayed with color coding to indicate current patient risk and any meaningful changes in risk (Army Medicine Public Affairs, 2013). BHDP data are also aggregated at various levels (e.g., military treatment facility [MTF], Army-wide) to assess treatment effectiveness and monitor the quality of BH care delivered. The Army tracks outcome measures, including response to treatment and remission of symptoms, as key indicators of improvement.

Army medicine has made a substantial investment in BHDP, and, after intensive and extended efforts to support its implementation, the system is now widely available in specialty BH settings. BHDP has been in operation since September 2013 in all 52 Army BH clinics (DoD, VA, and DHHS, 2016). As of July 2016, an average of 55,000–60,000 measures were completed each month in these clinics, for a total of more than 1.9 million measures collected by Army Behavioral Health. In 2013, the Assistant Secretary of Defense for Health Affairs mandated "measurement and documentation of clinical outcomes in mental health treatment [in all BH clinics] in Military Treatment Facilities" at the following intervals: "during initial evaluation and periodically until the termination of treatment in MH [mental health] treatment settings for patients diagnosed with: depression (PHQ-8), anxiety (GAD-7), and post-traumatic stress (PCL)" (Woodson, 2013). BHDP's implementation by other service branches was ongoing at the time of our study (DoD, VA, and DHHS, 2016). As of September 2016, BHDP had been implemented at 78 Navy clinics across 21 MTFs, and all identified Navy sites (134 clinics across 32 MTFs) were scheduled to have the system by March 2017. Targeted Air Force clinics had implemented BHDP, and 1,295 providers, counselors, psychological technicians, and administrative staff had been trained in its use.

These data, combined with other MHS health care utilization data, have the potential to inform decisions to improve the health and readiness of soldiers who receive BH care. BHDP offers data on soldier outcomes, providing a strategic opportu-

---

[1]   *DSM-5* refers to the *Diagnostic and Statistical Manual of Mental Disorders*, 5th ed.

nity to realize data-driven, measurement-based approaches to improving the health of soldiers who receive Army BH care.

Organization of This Report

This report focuses on active-component Army personnel who received a diagnosis of PTSD, depression, or anxiety in January–September 2016. We described demographic and service characteristics and utilization of care for soldiers with these BH conditions using administrative data as well as patterns of symptom scores for soldiers who received BH specialty care in the direct care system. Another analysis identified key factors (pretreatment and treatment) that were associated with changes in patient outcomes. Lastly, we characterized different trajectories of recovery based on symptom scores for soldiers who received Army BH specialty care.

Chapter Two describes our data sources, methods for the descriptive analyses, the creation of outcome variables and covariates, and the selection of the three samples (PTSD, depression, and anxiety) using data from December 2015–June 2017, as well as the multivariate analyses that we conducted to identify factors that predict changes in outcomes and different trajectories of recovery among active-component soldiers diagnosed with PTSD, depression, or anxiety who received Army BH care. Chapter Three examines patterns of treatment outcome monitoring for soldiers in the three samples and how outcome measures used by the Army compare with those used in NQF-endorsed measures. Chapter Four characterizes the soldiers who received a PTSD, depression, or anxiety disorder diagnosis and what MHS health care they used. It also assesses the representativeness of our samples. Chapter Five presents the results of our multivariate analyses to identify pretreatment variables (i.e., demographic and risk characteristics) and treatment variables that were associated with improved outcomes. Chapter Six identifies different trajectories of change for these soldiers, including predictors of different trajectories. Chapter Seven summarizes our main findings and offers recommendations for improving the quality of Army BH specialty care for PTSD, depression, and anxiety and for strengthening the Army's ongoing efforts to monitor and improve outcomes for these conditions. Appendix A contains the complete list of pretreatment and treatment variables evaluated in our prediction models. Appendix B provides detailed results from our multivariable logistic and linear regression models to identify predictors of outcomes.

CHAPTER TWO

Methods

Overview

In this chapter, we describe the methods used to conduct the analyses presented in this report. We describe our data sources; how we selected samples of soldiers with PTSD, depression, or anxiety for analyses; and how we defined symptom score outcomes. We also explain the statistical methods that we used to evaluate which demographic and risk characteristics and which aspects of treatment predicted treatment outcomes and describe how soldiers' symptoms change over time.

Data Sources

Table 2.1 provides a list of data files used in the analyses. These files included information about care delivered, symptom measures completed, and soldier demographic and service characteristics.

Cleaning Administrative Treatment Data

The administrative treatment data analyzed for this report included care provided to active-duty soldiers between December 1, 2015, and June 30, 2017.[1] These files contained records on all inpatient and outpatient health care provided by the MHS, including care provided in MTFs (direct care) and care provided by civilian providers and paid for by TRICARE (purchased care). We used extract files of administrative data for direct and purchased care created by the Defense Health Agency from the MHS Data Repository (Table 2.1). We linked and de-duplicated all records for each individual.[2]

---

[1] We also included care in the 12 months prior to study entry, which could have extended back to December 2014 for medical history and prior heath care utilization.

[2] Pharmacy Data Transaction Service (PDTS) files included only the scrambled Social Security number of the plan sponsor, the TRICARE policyholder. We expected that the majority of sponsors were the active-component service members themselves. However, to identify non-sponsor files, we cross-checked the PDTS with Virtual Storage Access Memory Military Health System Data Repository 2006 (VM6) beneficiary-level files to compare

Table 2.1
Data Files Used in the Analyses

Content	Data Files
Outpatient services delivered at MTFs (direct care)	Comprehensive Ambulatory Professional Encounter Record (CAPER)
Inpatient services delivered at MTFs (direct care)	Standard Inpatient Data Record (SIDR)
Provider services delivered outside of MTFs (purchased care)	TRICARE Encounter Data–Noninstitutional (TED-NI)
Facility services delivered outside of MTFs (purchased care)	TRICARE Encounter Data–Institutional (TED-I)
TRICARE eligibility and enrollment	Virtual Storage Access Memory Military Health System Data Repository 2006 (VM6) Beneficiary Level
TRICARE eligibility/active-duty status	Active-Duty Master File
Dispensed medication (direct and purchased care)	Pharmacy Data Transaction Services (PDTS)
Deployment history (September 2001– June 2017	Activation and Deployment File (Contingency Tracking System)
Additional transactions and dates of service entry and discharge	Active-Duty Transaction File
Symptom measures (e.g., PCL-5, PHQ-9, GAD-7)	BHDP

Preparing administrative data for use in selecting the analytic samples entailed extensive processing of direct care inpatient and outpatient stay records (SIDR and CAPER files) and purchased care provider and facility records (TED-NI and TED-I files) to ensure that encounters (i.e., outpatient visits, inpatient stays) were accurately counted.

To avoid double-counting, we eliminated duplicate records for the same inpatient stays. Because our analysis included inpatient care provided in acute care facilities, we excluded all nonacute care (i.e., rehabilitation care, residential/extended care, skilled nursing facility care, and home care) from the file of acute inpatient stays. We applied these rules to records in both the direct care inpatient file (i.e., SIDR) and the purchased care facility file (i.e., TED-I). Similar rules were applied to outpatient encounters. We counted multiple lines of data indicating the same provider specialty on the same date as a single outpatient visit for that specialty. We also counted multiple emergency department or ambulatory surgery records on the same date as a single outpatient visit, regardless of the number of providers or specialties recorded. Other

---

age and gender. We dropped cases that were not matches from our analyses (one age-category change to the next level during the measurement period was allowed).

than emergency department or ambulatory surgery, encounter records on the same day involving providers in different specialties (other than radiology) were counted as separate outpatient visits. Records indicating providers who generally provide ancillary services, such as general-duty nurses and corpsmen-technicians, were not counted as separate outpatient visits. We applied these rules to both the direct care outpatient file (i.e., CAPER) and the purchased care provider and facility files (i.e., TED-NI and TED-I). The detailed steps in this process, including variable names and codes, are documented elsewhere (Hepner, Sloss, et al., 2016).

Outcome Monitoring Data
Symptom Measures
Our analyses focused on symptom score data from three self-report measures, collected through BHDP: the PCL-5 for PTSD, the PHQ-9 for depression, and the GAD-7 for anxiety. The PCL-5 is a 20-item self-report measure that assesses past-month symptoms associated with PTSD (Blevins et al., 2015; Bovin et al., 2016; Weathers et al., 2013). Response options range from 0 (not at all) to 4 (extremely). The measure yields a score ranging from 0 to 80. The PCL-5 has been used in BHDP since October 2015.[3] Research suggests that a score cut point of 33 is indicative of PTSD, and a ten-point reduction in score indicates clinically meaningful improvement (Weathers et al., 2013). The Army has selected a PCL-5 score of 29 as the threshold to indicate a level of symptoms that suggests a need for further evaluation. These recommendations continue to evolve with the PCL-5's continued use.

Office of the Surgeon General/U.S. Army Medical Command Policy Memo 14-094 (Headquarters, U.S. Department of the Army, 2014) states, "Outcome measures will be routinely used for all individuals receiving PTSD treatment. The PTSD Checklist (PCL) will be used routinely before initiating PTSD treatment and at least on a monthly basis during the course of PTSD treatment." Since then, the Army has issued a similar requirement for providers to use the PCL at least every 30 days during treatment of PTSD and other trauma-related disorders (U.S. Army Medical Command, 2015).

The PHQ-9 is a nine-item depression symptom measure that aligns with the DSM-5 diagnostic criteria for major depressive disorder (Spitzer et al., 1999). Items assess frequency of symptoms in the past two weeks using response options ranging from 0 (not at all) to 3 (nearly every day). The total score ranges from 0 to 27. Total scores indicate the severity of depression symptoms: minimal (1–4), mild (5–9), moderate (10–14), moderately severe (15–19), or severe (20–27). A score of 10 or greater on the PHQ-9 has been suggested as a cut point for identifying cases of depression (Kroenke, Spitzer, and Williams, 2001). A PHQ-9 change score of five points or greater reflects

---

[3] Prior to October 2015, the Army used the PCL (based on DSM-IV diagnostic criteria) to monitor PTSD symptoms. In October 2015, the PCL-5 (based on updated DSM-5 criteria) replaced the PCL.

a clinically relevant change in individuals receiving depression treatment (Löwe et al., 2004). In 2015, the Army issued a requirement for providers to use the PHQ-9 at least every 30 days during treatment of major depression and other depressive disorders (U.S. Army Medical Command, 2015).

The GAD-7 is a seven-item symptom measure that assesses symptoms associated with anxiety (Spitzer et al., 2006). Response options range from 0 (not at all) to 3 (nearly every day), yielding a total score that can range from 0 to 21. Total scores of 5–9, 10–14, and 15–21 represent the range of scores for mild, moderate, and severe anxiety, respectively. A score of 10 or greater on the GAD-7 has been suggested as a cut point for identifying cases of generalized anxiety disorder (Spitzer et al., 2006). In 2015, Army issued a requirement for providers to use the GAD-7 at least every 30 days during treatment of anxiety disorders (U.S. Army Medical Command, 2015).

Symptom Score Outcome Measures

The PCL-5, PHQ-9, and GAD-7 are used to assess baseline severity of symptoms and track progress during treatment. In addition, the tools are used to document outcomes, defined as response to treatment and remission for those with initial scores above a defined threshold. Table 2.2 summarizes the requirements for soldier inclusion and the methodology for scoring using BHDP data for these measures that is currently in use by the Army to monitor these outcomes. Thresholds for response to treatment and remission are largely consistent with the available literature for these measures. Note that the populations defined as responding to treatment and in remission overlap for PTSD but are mutually exclusive for depression and anxiety.

Table 2.2
Army Scoring Methodology for Outcome Measures of Response and Remission

Outcome Measure	PTSD	Depression	Anxiety
Required elevated score for inclusion	PCL-5 score ≥29	PHQ-9 score ≥10	GAD-7 score ≥10
Response	≥10-point reduction from initial elevated PCL-5 score to last PCL-5 score	≥5-point reduction from initial elevated PHQ-9 score to last PHQ-9 score AND last PHQ-9 score >7	≥5-point reduction from initial elevated GAD-7 score to last GAD-7 score AND last GAD-7 score >7
Remission	Last PCL-5 score ≤22	≥5-point reduction from initial elevated PHQ-9 score to last PHQ-9 score AND last PHQ-9 score ≤7	≥5-point reduction from initial elevated GAD-7 score to last GAD-7 score AND last GAD-7 score ≤7

Preparing Symptom Measure Data for Analysis

BHDP includes several patient-reported measures and items, including the three symptom scores analyzed as outcomes (i.e., PCL-5, PHQ-9, GAD-7), along with other instruments, such as the 24-item Behavior and Symptom Identification Scale (BASIS-24) (Eisen et al., 2004) and the three-item Alcohol Use Disorders Identification Test–Concise (AUDIT-C) (Bush et al., 1998). We used total scores included in the data for each measure.[4] We linked each PCL-5, PHQ-9, and GAD-7 score and the date each measure was completed to the administrative data records of soldiers in our PTSD, depression, and anxiety samples.

Selecting Samples

We identified three samples of soldiers (PTSD, depression, and anxiety) who met a set of eligibility criteria. We used the criteria currently used by the Army to identify and monitor soldiers with these conditions for symptom response and remission. These criteria included the diagnosis codes defining the conditions, care setting, minimum symptom scores needed for sample inclusion, definition of a new treatment episode (NTE), and duration of observed follow-up care. Inclusion in a sample required having a diagnosis of PTSD, depression, or anxiety.[5] The diagnosis codes for PTSD included codes for acute, chronic, and unspecified PTSD. The diagnosis codes for depression included all codes for major depressive disorder but did not include dysthymia. The diagnosis codes for anxiety included agoraphobia, social phobia, panic disorder, generalized anxiety disorder, and other mixed and unspecified anxiety disorders but did not include specific phobias or obsessive-compulsive disorder. Members of the National Guard and reserves, retirees, and family members were not included in these analyses because these populations may be more likely to receive care outside of the MHS, which would not be captured in our analyses. The observation period during which we assessed symptom scores was a maximum of six months. Soldiers who may have later separated or deployed but were otherwise eligible for inclusion in our study were included in the samples. We used the following eligibility criteria to identify the PTSD, depression, and anxiety samples:

- *Active-duty soldier.* Every patient was required to be an active-duty soldier.

---

[4]   In general, measures with missing items are not included in the calculated scores. BASIS scoring allows for one missing item and employs a weighted substitution routine.

[5]   We used the following International Classification of Diseases, Tenth Revision, Clinical Modification (ICD-10-CM) codes to identify soldiers with a target condition:

- PTSD: F4310, F4311, and F4312
- depression: F320, F321, F322, F323, F324, F329, F330, F331, F332, F333, F339, and F3341
- anxiety disorders: F4000, F4001, F4002, F4010, F4011, F408, F409, F410, F411, F413, F418, and F419.

- *BH specialty visit for the target condition during the selection window.* Soldiers were required to have a direct care BH specialty visit with the target diagnosis (i.e., PTSD, depression, or anxiety) during the selection window (January–September 2016). In October 2015, the BHDP was altered to use the PCL-5 in place of the PCL. Specifying a selection window after October 2015 ensured consistent use of the PCL-5 during the entire study period and incorporated data for most recent care. The selection window also allowed for a six-month follow-up period after study entry. For this BH visit, the PTSD, depression, or anxiety International Classification of Diseases, Tenth Revision (ICD-10) diagnosis needed to be coded in the first (primary), second, or third position in the administrative data for the visit. At that visit, the soldier must have been seen by a physician, such as a psychiatrist (referred to as a Type 1 provider), or a psychologist or licensed clinical social worker (referred to as a Type 2 provider), and the visit type could not be a telephone consult or group appointment.
- *BH specialty visit qualifies as an NTE.* This BH specialty visit was also required to meet the requirements for a BH specialty care NTE. We defined an NTE as not having a previous BH specialty outpatient visit with the target diagnosis in any coded position (e.g., not having a PTSD diagnosis for those in the PTSD sample) in the six months prior to the first BH specialty visit during the sample selection window.
- *Completed a symptom measure with an elevated score close to the BH specialty visit for PTSD, depression, or anxiety.* Soldiers in the PTSD, depression, and anxiety samples were required to have completed a condition-related symptom measure within 30 days before or after the BH specialty visit (excluding scores with missing data). To be eligible, soldiers' symptom scores had to be at or above a specified threshold: a PCL-5 score of greater than or equal to 29 for PTSD, a PHQ-9 score of greater than or equal to 10 for depression, or a GAD-7 score of greater than or equal to 10 for anxiety.
- *Completed a follow-up symptom measure within one to six months.* Soldiers in the PTSD, depression, and anxiety samples were required to have completed a subsequent diagnosis-related symptom measure (e.g., PCL-5 for the PTSD sample) without any missing data one to six months after the first elevated symptom score.

Figure 2.1 shows the period during which soldiers in our samples could have an initial diagnosis ("Selection window for initial diagnosis") and the six-month periods for the initial elevated and last follow-up measure scores. The initial elevated score in the 30 days before and after the initial diagnosis (one of the criteria for inclusion in the sample) is referred to in the body of this report as the *initial* or *first* score. Since the first score could be 30 days prior to the diagnosis date (as early as December 2015), the last score could occur as early as January 2016.

Figure 2.1
Timing of Selection and Follow-Up of Samples

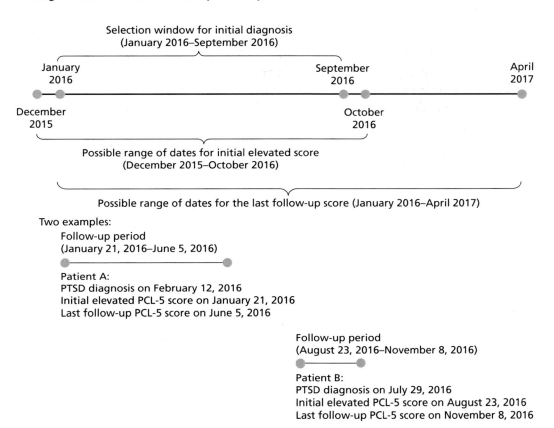

When considered together, these selection criteria mean that the three samples represent subsets of soldiers with PTSD, depression, or anxiety who completed at least two symptom measures and had an elevated symptom score within a month of the BH intake visit. However, the samples may not be representative of all service members with PTSD, depression, or anxiety, many of whom may not be captured by these selection criteria. Furthermore, the symptom scores of soldiers in the samples (e.g., those with initial and last follow-up scores) may not be representative of all soldiers with PTSD, depression, or anxiety or of all service members with a symptom score. As shown in Table 2.3, out of the soldiers in BH specialty care with a PTSD diagnosis in the first nine months of 2016, one-quarter (25 percent) were eligible for the PTSD sample (i.e., had an NTE of BH care, had an elevated PCL-5 score within 30 days of the start of the NTE, and completed another PCL-5 one to six months later). Similarly, out of the soldiers in BH specialty care with a depression diagnosis in 2016–2017, less than one-third (32 percent) were eligible for the depression sample. Out of the soldiers in BH specialty care with an anxiety diagnosis in 2016–2017, approximately one-quarter (24 percent) were eligible for the anxiety sample. Therefore, conclusions based on patterns of symp-

Table 2.3
Number of Soldiers in the Three Samples After Each Sample Requirement

Sample Requirement	PTSD % (n)	Depression % (n)	Anxiety % (n)
At least one direct care outpatient BH specialty visit[a] between January and September 2016 (n = 112,006)			
BH specialty visit with target diagnosis[b] and TRICARE Prime status	(n = 13,146)	(n = 11,906)	(n = 18,157)
No BH specialty visit with target diagnosis in the prior 6 months (new BH treatment episode)	52.3 (6,874)	57.3 (6,817)	64.5 (11,712)
Symptom score +/–30 days of target diagnosis date[c]	38.8 (5,098)	44.8 (5,338)	43.9 (7,977)

Elevated symptom score +/–30 days of new treatment episode start date[d]
  PTSD: PCL-5 score of ≥29
  Depression: PHQ-9 score of ≥10
  Anxiety: GAD-7 score of ≥10
	30.8 (4,046)	39.1 (4,656)	31.4 (5,704)

At least one follow-up symptom score 1 to 6 months after initial elevated score	24.8 (3,264)	31.9 (3,801)	23.6 (4,282)

[a] This visit was defined as a BH clinic encounter of any type for any diagnosis (coded as BF** in the Medical Expense and Performance Reporting System [MEPRS]).

[b] This visit was defined as a BH clinic visit (coded as BF** in MEPRS), provider type 1 or 2, not a telephone conference (TCON) or group (GRP) appointment. Target diagnoses for the PTSD, depression, and anxiety samples were PTSD, depression, or anxiety in diagnosis code position 1, 2, or 3.

[c] Symptom scores for the PTSD, depression, and anxiety samples were drawn from the PCL-5, PHQ-9, and GAD-7, respectively.

[d] If there was more than one elevated score, we used the first elevated score.

tom score data used for this study should be interpreted cautiously and may not apply to all soldiers with a diagnosis of one of the three conditions in 2016–2017.

Using these sample selection criteria, we identified 3,264 soldiers for the PTSD sample, 3,801 for the depression sample, and 4,282 for the anxiety disorder sample (Table 2.3). While the total number of soldiers receiving BH specialty care during January to September 2016 was 112,006, that number was significantly reduced by applying the sample inclusion criteria. The primary reason for exclusion was not having a target diagnosis code in position 1, 2, or 3. For this reason, 88 percent were excluded from the PTSD sample, 89 percent from the depression sample, and 83 percent from the anxiety sample. Less common reasons for exclusion were only having telephone conference or group encounters (5 percent) or no encounters with a Type 1 or 2 provider (3 percent). When all sample requirements were applied, 97 percent, 97 percent, and 96 percent of the 112,006 soldiers with any BH care during January to September 2016 were excluded from the PTSD, depression, and anxiety samples, respectively.

Therefore, these samples represent a small proportion of the soldiers with an encounter in BH specialty care during that time period.

The three samples were not selected to be mutually exclusive, so it was possible for a soldier to be in multiple samples. The overlap in samples is shown in Figure 2.2. The PTSD sample was the smallest of the three samples, with 3,264 soldiers, of whom 14 percent (n = 468 soldiers) were also in the depression sample, 16 percent were also in the anxiety sample (n = 521), and 6 percent were in all three samples (n = 191). The depression sample was next in size with 3,801 soldiers, of whom 12 percent were also in the PTSD sample (n = 468), 17 percent were also in the anxiety sample (n = 633), and 5 percent were in all three samples (n = 191). The anxiety sample was the largest with 4,282 soldiers, of whom 12 percent were also in the PTSD sample (n = 521), 15 percent were also in the depression sample (n = 633), and 4 percent were in all three samples (n = 191). Note that the rates of overlap among these samples were driven by the selection approach (including requiring two scores for the target diagnosis) and that the actual rate of comorbidity among these diagnoses is higher.

Figure 2.2
Overlap of the PTSD, Depression, and Anxiety Samples

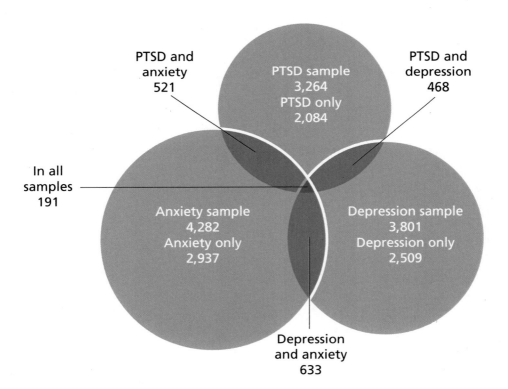

Predictors of Behavioral Health Treatment Outcomes

We developed several patient and treatment variables that were potential predictors of BH treatment outcomes in patients with PTSD, depression, or anxiety. Our work was informed by considering the literature to determine what variables might be predictors of outcomes for our target conditions. Some of the suggested variables included number and concentration of psychotherapy sessions, group versus individual psychotherapy, type of psychotherapy provided, and level of pretreatment severity (Cuijpers et al., 2013; Haagen et al., 2015; Keefe et al., 2014). We then limited the variables we considered to those available in administrative data and the BHDP. We grouped the predictors into two categories: pretreatment variables (e.g., demographic characteristics, military service, comorbid diagnoses and symptoms, use of health care before the initial elevated score) and treatment variables (e.g., psychotherapy, individual therapy, group therapy, provider, evaluation and management [E&M] visits, total visits, medications). Using this process, we defined a total of 57 pretreatment variables and 84 treatment variables (including three covariates that captured the timing of the initial score relative to the intake visit). Examples of pretreatment and treatment variables that we included in the multivariate models are shown in Table 2.4. A complete list of all variables can be found in Appendix A.

Analyses

In this section, we describe our analytic approach. We restricted all analyses of symptom measure data to those completed by soldiers between December 2015 and April 2017.[6]

Understanding BHDP Implementation and Army Outcome Measures

The focus of our study was to identify predictors of soldier outcomes using symptom measures collected through BHDP, so we first sought to understand patterns of BHDP measure completion. We conducted our analyses using the three selected samples: 3,284 soldiers diagnosed with PTSD, 3,801 diagnosed with depression, and 4,482 diagnosed with anxiety. These analyses focused on describing how and when measures specific to PTSD, depression, and anxiety symptoms were completed, including the length of time between a soldier's initial score and final follow-up score, the frequency with which soldiers completed the outcome measures, and the relationship between the number of BH specialty visits that soldiers received and the number of scores in their administrative files. We conducted analyses to describe the relationship between the number of completed symptom measures and the number of BH specialty visits during

---

[6] Symptom data used to calculate outcomes based on NQF-endorsed measures of depression response and remission in Chapter Three used BHDP scores through June 2017.

Table 2.4
Examples of Pretreatment and Treatment Variables Included in Models

Example Variable	Variable Description
Pretreatment Variables:	
Marital status	Marital status at initial elevated score [Married; divorced; separated; never married]
Total deployments	Total number of deployments at initial elevated score
General distress (BASIS score)	Behavior and Symptom Identification Scale (BASIS), 30 days prior to 1 week after initial elevated score
Function, personal/social (WRAIR PSF score)	Walter Reed Functional Impairment Scale, personal/social functioning score
Anxiety, past history	Diagnosis of anxiety in >30 days to 12 months prior to initial elevated score
MH outpatient visits	Number of outpatient mental health encounters in >30 days to 12 months prior to initial elevated score
Time Covariates:	
Total days between first-last scores	Number of days between initial elevated and last scores
Treatment Variables:	
Any evidence-based therapy	Flag for at least 1 session with evidence-based therapy
Therapeutic Alliance Questionnaire score	Last DoD/VA Therapeutic Alliance Questionnaire score using a 3-item scale developed by Army
E&M, all care, primary diagnosis	Number of evaluation and management visits, direct care and purchased care: target condition primary diagnosis
Group therapy visits, direct care, primary/secondary diagnosis, per month, categorical	Categorical number of group therapy sessions, direct care, per month: target condition diagnosis in any position [0 visits; >0 to <3 visits; 3 to ≤4 visits; >4 visits]
Individual therapy visits, direct care, primary diagnosis, per month	Number of individual therapy sessions, direct care per month: target condition primary diagnosis
3+ visits, primary/secondary diagnosis, type 1 provider	Flag for dosage met: 3+ visits in 90 days after intake (BF clinic, not TCON), target condition diagnosis in any position, type 1 provider: regardless of timing of first score relative to intake
Any MH purchased care	Flag for any purchased care for any mental health diagnosis
Benzodiazepine, days' supply, categorical	Categorical benzodiazepine days' supply dispensed [0 days; 1–30 days; >30 days]

NOTE: BF = MEPRS code (second level) for behavioral health clinic; WRAIR = Walter Reed Army Institute of Research; PSF = personal/social function.

the six months after the initial score.[7] We also examined the Army's use of BHDP data to compute and monitor rates of response and remission for the three target conditions. Outside of the MHS, depression response and remission outcomes are monitored with an NQF-endorsed measure that is used by Medicare, Medicaid, and some commercial health plans and has been added to the 2017 Healthcare Effectiveness Data and Information Set (HEDIS). Therefore, we also examined the implications of the Army's approach to monitoring depression outcomes compared with the NQF measure's methodology. Results of these analyses are presented in Chapter Three.

Representativeness of Soldiers in Samples

We assessed the representativeness of each of the samples (excluding cases with missing data) for the pretreatment variables. Because of missing data on the predictor variables, the sizes of the samples included in the multivariate models were as follows: 1,528 for PTSD, 1,849 for depression, and 2,592 for anxiety. We assessed representativeness by comparing the demographic and service characteristics and health care utilization of soldiers in the samples with those of a broader group of soldiers who were excluded during the selection process. Specifically, we identified a comparison group of soldiers with at least one direct care BH specialty visit for the target diagnosis (e.g., PTSD) but who were excluded from the respective sample.[8] We evaluated how each sample differed from the broader one-visit group in terms of demographic characteristics (gender, age, and race/ethnicity), service characteristics (pay grade and deployment history), health care utilization characteristics (outpatient visits [total and for MH diagnoses]), and the rate of co-occurring conditions. For these analyses, we report descriptive statistics, including frequency counts, percentages, and medians. We performed chi-square (for categorical variables) and t-tests (for continuous variables) to examine whether these variables differed significantly between each sample and between the soldiers in our samples and the soldiers who were excluded. Results of these analyses are presented in Chapter Four.

Identifying Predictors of Symptom Change

Two sets of analyses assessed the degree of association between the predictors and various diagnostic outcomes. First, we conducted analyses to identify predictors of outcome improvement for soldiers with PTSD, depression, or anxiety—defined as the change in outcome score from the initial to the last observed outcome score (i.e., last minus initial score). We also conducted exploratory analyses to characterize different

---

[7]   BH specialty visits were restricted to direct care and identified on the basis of the MEPRS2 (second-level MEPRS) variable coded as BF in the CAPER file and excluded TCON visits.

[8]   The comparison group of soldiers with at least one direct care BH specialty visit for the target condition was defined as having at least one direct care BH specialty visit with the target condition diagnosis (in position 1–3), with provider type 1 or 2, that was other than a TCON or group appointment.

trajectories of improvement in scores for soldiers who received Army BH specialty care, taking into account all the changes observed over time.

Identifying Predictors of Outcome Improvement

Because we considered a large number of potential predictors, we conducted a systematic variable selection process to arrive at a more concise set of predictors. Variable selection (e.g., Draper and Smith, 1981; Hocking, 1976) included an assessment of the distribution of the predictors to ensure that they had adequate variability, a bivariate analysis to identify variables that were potentially associated with the outcomes, and a grouped multivariate analysis within different conceptual groups of variables to evaluate collinearity between these potential variables. The goal of this multistep process was to develop a parsimonious model in which only the necessary variables were tested for association with the outcomes. The primary model building was conducted with the continuous change in symptom score as the outcome variable and a set of predictor variables, which included the initial symptom score, that we analyzed using linear regression. We systematically applied a set of selection criteria to the potential predictors for each condition (PTSD, depression, and anxiety) using a multistep process (shown in Figure 2.3). To manage the large number of potential predictor variables, we split them into two sets: pretreatment variables (demographic, military service, and use of health care before the initial score) and treatment variables related to the behavioral health care provided for the target condition after the initial symptom score. We used the same approach to select a subset of pretreatment variables and a subset of the treatment variables.

Step 1 for Pretreatment Variables

In step 1, we reviewed information about "missingness" and variability for each patient variable (Figure 2.3). We dropped variables with more than 20 percent of values missing from the set of predictors because the soldiers with missing values would have to be excluded from the model, thereby reducing the effective sample size. We also dropped categorical variables for which almost all study participants were in one category and all the other categories captured less than 10 percent of the sample. For example, for the variable "having a personality disorder," only 1 percent of the sample had a diagnosis of the disorder and 99 percent did not, indicating low variability. Thus, this variable was not adequate for inclusion as a covariate. For continuous variables, we dropped those that had no variability.

Step 2 for Pretreatment Variables

In step 2, we conducted a set of bivariate analyses to assess the magnitude and direction of the relationship between each predictor variable and the continuous outcome variable (as shown in Figure 2.3). For all final models tested, we controlled for initial symptom scores; as such, the models with a change in outcome score controlling for the initial score were equivalent to the models with the last outcome controlling for

Figure 2.3
Selection of Variables for Multivariate Models to Predict Outcomes of BH Treatment

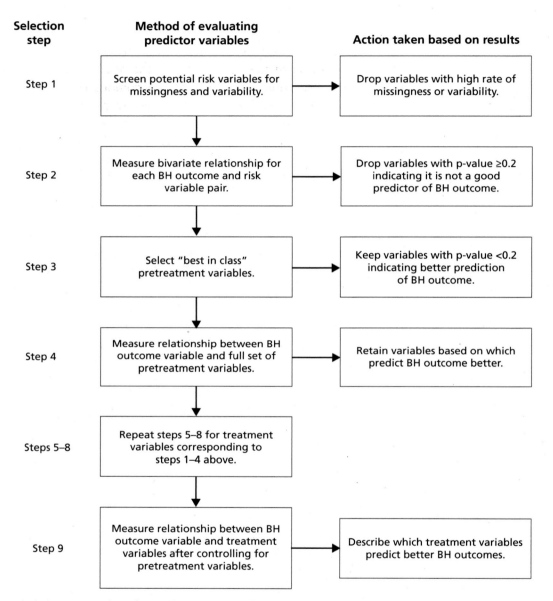

Selection step	Method of evaluating predictor variables	Action taken based on results
Step 1	Screen potential risk variables for missingness and variability.	Drop variables with high rate of missingness or variability.
Step 2	Measure bivariate relationship for each BH outcome and risk variable pair.	Drop variables with p-value ≥0.2 indicating it is not a good predictor of BH outcome.
Step 3	Select "best in class" pretreatment variables.	Keep variables with p-value <0.2 indicating better prediction of BH outcome.
Step 4	Measure relationship between BH outcome variable and full set of pretreatment variables.	Retain variables based on which predict BH outcome better.
Steps 5–8	Repeat steps 5–8 for treatment variables corresponding to steps 1–4 above.	
Step 9	Measure relationship between BH outcome variable and treatment variables after controlling for pretreatment variables.	Describe which treatment variables predict better BH outcomes.

NOTE: Steps were also informed by the literature on predictors of outcome, and selection favored variables that were considered actionable (i.e., variables that could be adjusted by the Army through quality improvement efforts).

initial score. For this reason, in this step, we sought to retain any variable possibly related to the last symptom score. We retained a few variables commonly used in the literature for these types of prediction models, regardless of their bivariate association with the outcomes. These variables included the soldier's age, race/ethnicity, sex, marital status, pay grade, and number of deployments. Next, we used t-tests from the linear models to determine association of the outcome with the other potential predictor variables when assessing continuous variables and dichotomous variables. For categorical variables with more than two levels, we used an F-test from the analysis of variance (ANOVA). If the test of significance (p-value) was less than 0.10, we retained predictors for the next stage. If the p-value was between 0.10 and 0.20, we discussed and decided whether to retain the variable in the analysis based on its clinical importance and our expert opinion. This additional flexibility allowed us to retain variables for further evaluation that we believed could be clinically important. If the p-value exceeded 0.20, we dropped the predictor before the next stage. We repeated the set of bivariate analyses with the two secondary outcome variables of interest, the response and remission outcomes.

Step 3 for Pretreatment Variables

Because similar variables are likely to be highly correlated, in step 3, we grouped the predictor variables by content (e.g., demographic characteristics, comorbid conditions or symptoms, prior treatment) and entered them as groups into mini-multivariate models to assess multicollinearity within groups (see Figure 2.3). We again evaluated predictors using t-tests or F-tests. If the level of association for a predictor variable within a group showed a p-value of less than 0.10, we retained the predictor for the next stage. If the p-value was between 0.10 and 0.20, we evaluated whether to retain the variable in the analysis based on its clinical importance and our expert opinion. This allowed us to retain variables with clinical relevance that might have a very weak bivariate association with the outcomes. If such variables were still not relevant, they would be dropped in the next step (described below). If the p-value exceeded 0.20, we dropped the predictor before the next stage because information provided by such predictors could be accounted for by the retained predictors. In a few cases, if two predictor variables were correlated and there was consensus that one could be more actionable for quality improvement, based on our team's judgment, we retained the more actionable variable instead of the other variable irrespective of the association inference detected by the within-group multivariate model. For example, we retained variables that allowed us to assess direct care visits received for the target diagnosis coded in the first position and dropped variables that represented all care (i.e., direct and purchased care) because the Army may have more influence over direct care visits than purchased care visits. Furthermore, when multiple variables were similar or correlated, we retained variables assessing care for the target diagnosis (PTSD, depression, or anxiety) over variables that assessed care for the target diagnosis in *any* position or *any* BH diagnosis.

Step 4 for Pretreatment Variables

In step 4, we ran multivariate models with the continuous change in symptom score variable as the outcome and all patient variables retained from steps 1–3 as predictors (see Figure 2.3). We used a 0.05 significance level for inference in this multivariate model. The results of these step 4 models, including the model parameters, are presented in Appendix B. Based on similar results from the models for the three conditions, we concluded that a consistent set of patient variables should be included in all models.

Steps 5 Through 8 for Treatment Variables

We followed the same process of selecting predictor variables from the treatment set, repeating steps 1–4 to identify the subset of treatment variables that were associated with symptom score outcomes. We repeated the methods used in steps 1–4 for the pretreatment variables in steps 5–8 for the treatment variables.

Step 9 for Pretreatment and Treatment Variables

In step 9, we conducted multivariate models with the continuous symptom score as the outcome (considered the primary outcome) and all pretreatment and treatment variables that retained as predictors from the selection processes (steps 1–8) (see Figure 2.3). We identified two necessary time-related covariates that we controlled for in the final step 9 models. First, some soldiers had an initial score *after* their visit that would be considered the beginning of their NTE. Care received between their initial visit and the initial score could have an impact on their initial score. Second, soldiers had varying time periods between their initial score and their last score, giving them varying opportunities to receive treatment and improve. Therefore, we included whether the initial score was measured after the initial (intake) visit and the number of days from initial score to the last follow-up score. The results of these models are presented in Chapter Five.

As supplementary analyses, we used logistic regression to examine the dichotomous symptom score variables (i.e., response to treatment and remission, the secondary outcomes) using the predictor variables retained in each final (i.e., step 9) continuous outcome models.

Identifying Symptom Score Trajectories

In addition to the analysis of change scores from initial to last score (discussed in the previous section), we conducted a trajectory analysis using a linear growth curve method to assess the incremental changes that occurred from visit to visit. Unlike the previous analysis in step 9, this analysis also assumes a linear association between the outcomes and time, and its goal is to detect different classes (or groups) of soldiers depending on how their outcomes change over time. For this analysis, we grouped soldiers based on their likelihood of having a specific type of outcome improvement trajectory over time. We examined patterns of PTSD, depression, and anxiety symptom scores over time to characterize the different symptom trajectories (i.e., patterns of change over time). To retain as many soldiers as possible in the trajectory analysis, we included the samples of soldiers with each diagnosis, regardless of missing predictor variables. However, to ensure that we had enough information on each soldier to assess his or her trajectory, we restricted these analyses to soldiers with at least three symptom scores. The resulting sample sizes were 2,779 for PTSD, 3,394 for depression, and 3,601 for anxiety.

We conducted latent class analyses (LCAs) (Goodman, 1974), controlling for such demographic variables as the soldier's age, race/ethnicity, sex, marital status, pay grade, and number of deployments to identify empirically driven recovery trajectories of improvement. With the different number of observed symptom scores from one soldier to the next, interpretation from a non-linear LCA can be complex, and, therefore, only linear latent class models were used. An LCA hypothesizes that an individual's patterns in change over time can be accounted for by a small number of mutually exclusive groups (i.e., classes). For example, one group of soldiers could show improvement in symptoms over time while another group does not show improvement. Analytically, for a fixed number of trajectories, the LCA model estimates the optimal assignment of soldiers to each trajectory group so that members of a specific group have a similar trajectory of improvement and initial symptom score (after controlling for covariates). For each sample (PTSD, depression, and anxiety), we allowed up to seven trajectories (i.e., classes), hypothesizing that this would be the maximum number observed in the data (and we could have extended that maximum number if analyses suggest poor model fit). We fit a latent class model for each of the possible groups. To select the best-fitting model, we used the Bayesian Information Criterion (Raftery, 1993) and the Lo-Mendell-Rubin adjusted likelihood ratio test (Lo, Mendell, and Rubin, 2001), per the recommendations of Nylund and colleagues (Nylund, Asparouhov, and Muthén, 2007). Models with lower Bayesian Information Criterions are considered better fitting than those with higher values (Hagenaars and McCutcheon, 2002). When the model results suggested that outliers were forming their own very small class, we dropped these outliers and reran the models. The best-fitting model is reported as a plot of different trajectories. For each model, we estimated the probability of a soldier belonging to a specific latent trajectory group and then classified soldiers as being in the group that they had the highest probability of belonging. We then conducted chi-square tests and one-way ANOVAs to identify treatment variables retained in the selection of treatment variables for the multivariate models (step 8) that were associated with belonging to a specific trajectory group. The results of the symptom score trajectory analyses are presented in Chapter Six.

Samples for Analysis

We describe results in Chapters Three though Six. The types of analyses performed and the related inclusion criteria used, resulted in varying sample sizes across these analyses. For clarity, in Table 2.5 we summarize details of the varying sample sizes by chapter. We begin with Chapter Three to highlight background information about the Army's implementation of monitoring outcomes for PTSD, depression, and anxiety. The results of the multivariate analyses are presented in Chapter Five, but as an introduction to those results, we provide descriptive data about the multivariate analytic samples in Chapter Four.

Table 2.5
Summary of Samples Used in Analyses

			N		
Chapter	Sample	Sample Description	PTSD	Depression	Anxiety
Three	Outcome monitoring	Based on soldiers meeting inclusion criteria for Army outcome monitoring (Table 2.3) Sample used to describe Army implementation of outcome measures	3,264	3,801	4.262
Four	Multivariate analysis	Based on sample used in multivariate analyses (Chapter Five) Sample size reduction related to loss of individuals with missing variable values Sample used in this chapter to describe • demographics • utilization • comorbidities • symptom severity • comparison to those in BH care with same diagnosis but not meeting inclusion criteria for analysis	1,528	1,849	2,592
Five	Multivariate analysis	Sample used in multivariable analyses Sample used to identify pretreatment and treatment predictors	1,528	1,849	2,592
Six	Trajectory analysis	Sample used to identify trajectories of symptom change Sample size reduction related to inclusion criterion requiring at least 3 symptom scores	2,779	3,394	3,601

CHAPTER THREE

Implementation of Treatment Outcome Monitoring and the Army's Outcome Measures

In this chapter, we describe the patterns of outcome monitoring within BHDP to gauge implementation and use of the system. Subsequently, we describe the rates of achieving response to treatment and remission for PTSD, depression, and anxiety using the Army's methodology for monitoring these outcomes. We also compare this methodology with the NQF's approach to defining response and remission measures for individuals with depression. For these analyses, we use the outcome monitoring sample, as described in Chapter Two. Based on our analyses, key findings in this chapter include the following:

- The frequency of symptom measures administered over time varied, but most soldiers had at least three months between initial and last symptom scores.
- Soldiers with longer follow-up periods had more symptom scores recorded.
- Soldiers with more BH visits had more symptom scores recorded.
- Rates of response or remission based on Army methodology were 35 percent for PTSD, 45 percent for depression, and 41 percent for anxiety.
- Differences between the Army methodology for computing depression response and remission measures and the NQF-endorsed measures make comparison between Army and civilian care difficult.

Patterns of Outcome Monitoring

In this section, we describe the patterns of outcome monitoring for soldiers who received BH care who had diagnoses of PTSD, depression, or anxiety. These analyses provide information that may guide the Army's continued BHDP implementation efforts in BH specialty clinics. These results can also aid in interpreting the findings discussed elsewhere in this report, such as highlighting when follow-ups occurred for soldiers included in analyses.

Timing of Last Follow-Up Score

Repeated administrations of symptom measures allow monitoring of symptom change over time, which is particularly useful when assessing a patient's response to treatment. We examined the length of time between each soldier's initial elevated score and final follow-up score. The observation period included up to six months after the initial score, based on the sample selection criteria; thus, these results do not include measures completed after six months. It is possible that soldiers continued to improve after the last score, which would not be included in our data if it was longer than six months later. While six months is a relatively short time, an NQF-endorsed measure of depression outcome assesses improvement in the last follow-up scores within four to eight months, indicating a possibility of improvement within that shorter time frame of four months (NQF, 2018), and some patients reach remission of depression within six months (Angstman, Rohrer, and Rasmussen, 2012). Table 3.1 describes the number of days between first and last symptom measure scores for each of the three samples: soldiers receiving BH treatment who had a diagnosis of PTSD (PCL-5), soldiers receiving BH treatment who had a diagnosis of depression (PHQ-9), and soldiers receiving BH treatment who had a diagnosis of anxiety (GAD-7).

We observed similar patterns across the three samples. Nearly half of the PTSD and depression samples (48 percent and 47 percent, respectively) had their last score almost six months (i.e., 151–180 days) after the initial score. Somewhat fewer in the anxiety sample (41 percent) had this length of follow-up. About one-third had their follow-up scores between three and five months after the initial score (32 percent for PTSD, 31 percent for depression, and 32 percent for anxiety). However, between 21 and 27 percent of soldiers in each of the samples had their last score within 31–90 days of the initial score: 21 percent for PTSD, 22 percent for depression, and 27 percent for anxiety. Although the majority of soldiers in each of the three samples had at least three months between the initial and last score, soldiers with less time between their initial and last scores may be less likely to show clinically significant change, as there may be less opportunity to receive adequate treatment in that period.

Table 3.1
Percentage of Soldiers in Outcome Monitoring Samples, by Days Between Initial and Last Follow-Up Scores, 2016–2017

Days Between Initial and Last Scores	PTSD (n = 3,264) % (n)	Depression (n = 3,801) % (n)	Anxiety (n = 4,282) % (n)
31–60 days	7.1 (231)	8.9 (339)	10.6 (453)
61–90 days	13.7 (446)	12.9 (492)	15.9 (682)
91–120 days	11.8 (384)	12.8 (486)	13.2 (563)
121–150 days	20.0 (653)	18.1 (689)	19.0 (815)
151–180 days	47.5 (1,550)	47.2 (1,795)	41.3 (1,769)

A sizable minority of soldiers had their last score within 90 days of their initial score, but the reasons for this pattern are not clear. Soldiers may be seen for a BH specialty visit but may not have a measure administered during their visit. Alternatively, a soldier may not return to BH specialty care, perhaps because treatment was completed or discontinued. We also examined whether soldiers received at least one BH specialty care visit after their last score (within six months after their initial score). Table 3.2 shows that more than half of soldiers received a BH visit *after* their last symptom score. For each sample, almost half to three-fifths of soldiers who received their initial and last follow-up score within five months received at least one BH care specialty visit after the last score. Soldiers who had five to six months in between their initial and last score appeared less likely to receive at least one additional care visit, though the period remaining was short. These results suggest that some soldiers may receive BH visits without being administered symptom measures.

Frequency of Outcome Monitoring

The number of scores for each soldier can provide information about how BH providers may be using measure scores to inform treatment. These results also indicate how well these data support an examination of different longitudinal trajectories of change, which are typically more robust when integrating three or more scores. Table 3.3 shows the number of symptom scores reported within each soldier's follow-up period (i.e., from initial to last symptom score within one to six months).

Numbers of symptom scores in the one to six months of follow-up varied by sample for soldiers receiving BH care that had a diagnosis of PTSD, depression, or anxiety. Soldiers in the PTSD sample were the most likely to receive 10 or more PCL-5 scores. Nearly a quarter (24 percent) had ten or more scores; more than half (53 percent) had more than five scores. Soldiers in the depression sample had a similar pattern of PHQ-9 scores. Twenty percent had ten or more scores, and more than half (55 per-

Table 3.2
Percentage of Soldiers in Outcome Monitoring Samples with a BH Visit After Last Score, by Days Between Initial and Last Scores, 2016–2017

Days Between Initial and Last Scores	Soldiers with One or More BH Visits After Last Symptom Score		
	PTSD (n = 3,264) % (n)	Depression (n = 3,801) % (n)	Anxiety (n = 4,282) % (n)
31–60 days	61.9 (143)	55.8 (189)	57.2 (259)
61–90 days	64.6 (288)	59.6 (293)	61.7 (421)
91–120 days	56.3 (216)	47.3 (230)	49.2 (277)
121–150 days	61.9 (404)	57.2 (394)	57.4 (468)
151–180 days	39.1 (606)	37.9 (680)	38.2 (676)

Table 3.3
Percentage of Soldiers in Outcome Monitoring Samples, by Number of Symptom Scores in Their Follow-Up Period, 2016–2017

Number of Scores Within Each Soldier's Follow-Up Period	PTSD (n = 3,264) % (n)	Depression (n = 3,801) % (n)	Anxiety (n = 4,282) % (n)
2–3	27.1 (885)	23.1 (877)	32.4 (1,386)
4–5	19.7 (644)	22.2 (843)	23.7 (1,014)
6–7	15.4 (501)	19.6 (744)	17.8 (760)
8–9	13.7 (446)	15.1 (575)	11.8 (507)
10 or more	24.1 (788)	20.1 (762)	14.4 (615)

NOTES: The length of the follow-up period is the time between first and last scores. This varies by soldier and could be from 31 to 180 days after the initial score.

cent) had more than five scores. Soldiers in the anxiety sample were the least likely to receive multiple and frequent GAD-7 scores. Only 14 percent had ten or more scores; less than half had more than five scores. The Army's monitoring of anxiety symptoms was implemented after monitoring for PTSD and depression, so these results could reflect differing stages of implementation.

These findings show that the number of scores varied substantially both within each of the three samples and across the three samples. One limitation of these analyses is that it is unclear what an adequate number of scores would be for each soldier, as the length of time between first and last scores varies by soldier (e.g., one month for some, six months for others). Therefore, we also conducted analyses to examine the number of scores by length of time between the first and last score (see Figures 3.1–3.3). As expected, these analyses suggested that soldiers with lengthier periods between their first and last scores had more scores overall. Specifically, Figure 3.1 shows that soldiers in the PTSD sample who had longer periods between their first and last PCL-5 scores were more likely to receive more frequent scores. For example, the majority (61 percent) of those whose first and last scores were between five and six months apart received eight or more scores, while the majority (94 percent) of those with follow-up periods between one and two months received five or fewer scores.

We observed similar patterns for the depression sample (see Figure 3.2). For example, more than one-third of soldiers whose first and last PHQ-9 scores were between five and six months apart received ten or more scores, while only 9 percent received just two or three scores. More than half (59 percent) of those whose first and last scores were between one and two months apart received two or three scores, while none received ten or more scores.

Finally, we observed similar patterns for soldiers in the anxiety sample (see Figure 3.3). For example, 29 percent of those whose first and last GAD-7 scores were

Figure 3.1
Number of PCL-5 Scores, by Days of Follow-Up for Soldiers in the PTSD Outcome Monitoring Sample (n = 3,264), 2016–2017

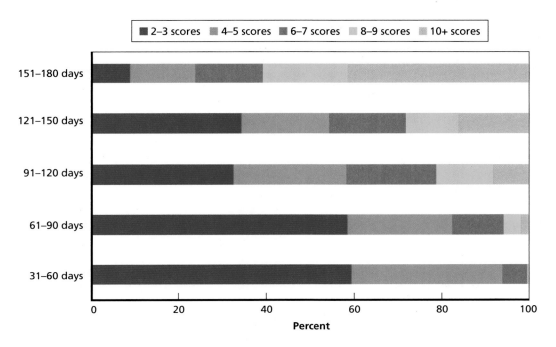

between five and six months apart received ten or more scores, while only 12 percent received just two or three scores. More than three-fifths (68 percent) of those whose first and last scores were between one and two months apart received two or three scores, while none received ten or more scores.

In summary, a longer length of time between first and last scores was associated with a higher number of scores, a finding that was consistent across our samples. This is a promising indicator of widespread BHDP implementation in Army BH specialty care. However, a sizable proportion of soldiers within each sample had very few scores, despite being in care for multiple months.

Relationship Between Frequency of Outcome Monitoring and BH Specialty Visits

Our previous analyses examined the number of scores in a soldier's record by the length of time between the first and last scores. Yet the number of BH specialty visits that soldiers received during this period varied. We also examined the relationship between the number of BH specialty visits and the number of measure scores for each sample (see Figures 3.4–3.6). Given that measures are largely administered during BH visits, it would be unlikely for soldiers to have more scores than BH visits. For the PTSD sample, a clear pattern emerged showing that soldiers who received more BH care visits had more scores, and soldiers with fewer BH care specialty visits had fewer scores (see

Figure 3.2
**Number of PHQ-9 Scores, by Days of Follow-Up for Soldiers in the Depression Outcome
Monitoring Sample (n = 3,801), 2016–2017**

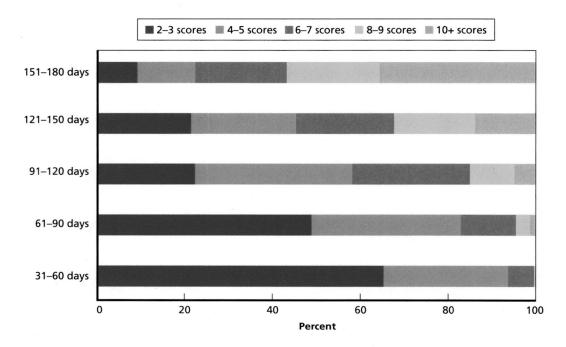

Figure 3.4). For example, the majority (64 percent) of those with 16 or more BH care visits had eight or more scores, while the majority (72 percent) of those with one to five BH visits had two or three scores.

A similar pattern emerged for the depression sample (see Figure 3.5): Soldiers who received more BH care visits had more scores, and soldiers with fewer BH care specialty visits had fewer scores. For example, the majority (65 percent) receiving 16 or more visits had eight or more scores, while almost three-quarters (73 percent) of soldiers with one to five BH visits had two or three PHQ-9 scores.

We observed this pattern again in the anxiety sample (see Figure 3.6). More than half (57 percent) of those receiving 16 or more visits had eight or more scores, while more than three-quarters (76 percent) of soldiers with one to five BH visits had two or three GAD-7 scores. However, compared with those in the PTSD and depression samples, nearly double the percentage of those with 16 or more visits for anxiety had only two or three scores (16 percent).

In summary, as the number of BH visits increased, the number of symptom scores increased in all three samples. These analyses are a promising indicator that BHDP implementation is working well, although there is some room for improvement. There were many soldiers who had lengthy periods between their first and last scores or who received multiple BH visits but had only a few scores. This was more apparent for those

Figure 3.3
Number of GAD-7 Scores, by Days of Follow-Up for Soldiers in the Anxiety Outcome Monitoring Sample (n = 4,282), 2016–2017

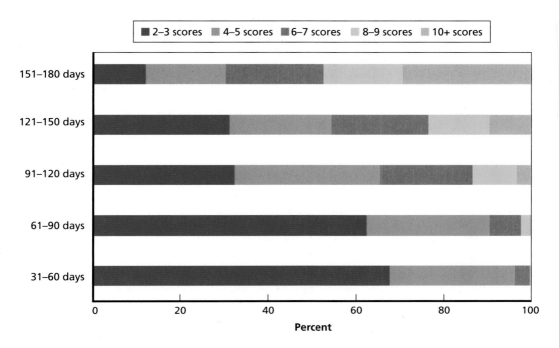

with a diagnosis of anxiety than for those with a diagnosis of PTSD or depression. These findings suggest that more consistent and repeated use of symptom measures is likely needed for those in longer-term care so that symptom change can be effectively monitored. While the Army recommends measuring symptoms every 30 days while in treatment, it was not within the scope of this project to analyze compliance with that recommendation.

Army Outcome Measures

In this section, we compare two approaches to defining outcome measures using BHDP data. The definitions used in the technical specifications for outcome measures impact the resulting performance rates. For example, the technical specifications, such as selecting the denominator and defining the follow-up period, determine which individuals are eligible for inclusion in the measure. First, we describe the Army's current methods of monitoring outcomes (response to treatment and remission) for PTSD, depression, and anxiety. Then, we compare the Army's outcome measures for depression with the NQF-endorsed outcome measures for depression.

Figure 3.4
Percentage of Soldiers in the PTSD Outcome Monitoring Sample (n = 3,264) with Specified Number of PCL-5 Scores, by Number of BH Specialty Visits in Direct Care, 2016–2017

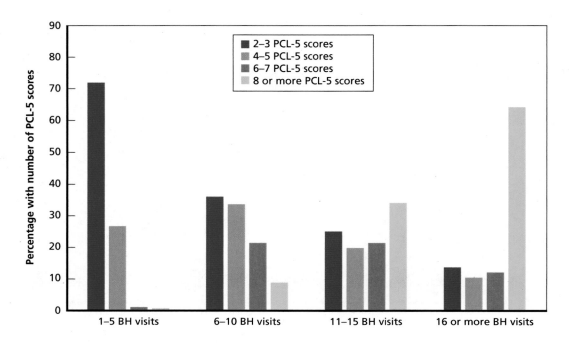

Army Outcomes for Response and Remission

The specifications for the response and remission scores for the three target conditions using the Army methodology are summarized in Table 2.2 in Chapter Two. The performance rates on these outcome measures may be reported for response, remission, or having achieved either response or remission. *Response*, an indicator of symptom improvement, is defined by the Army methodology for depression and anxiety as a five-point drop in score, but with a last score that remains at 8 or higher, suggesting some remaining symptomatology. Response for PTSD is defined as at least a 10-point reduction in score. *Remission* for depression and anxiety is defined as a five-point drop in score and a last score of 7 or less, suggesting remission of symptoms (or recovery). Remission for PTSD is defined as a last score of 22 or lower. Higher rates of response and remission indicate better outcomes. Table 3.4 shows the outcome results for the three diagnoses using the Army methodology and the outcomes monitoring sample. Note that the definitions of *response* and *remission* used by the Army result in response and remission populations that are exclusive for depression and anxiety but overlap for PTSD. Rates of "response or remission" were highest for depression (45 percent), followed by anxiety (41 percent) and PTSD (35 percent). Among the diagnoses, the rate of response was highest for PTSD (35 percent), and the rate of remission was highest for anxiety (27 percent).

Figure 3.5
Percentage of Soldiers in the Depression Outcome Monitoring Sample (n = 3,801) with Specified Number of PHQ-9 Scores, by Number of BH Specialty Visits in Direct Care, 2016–2017

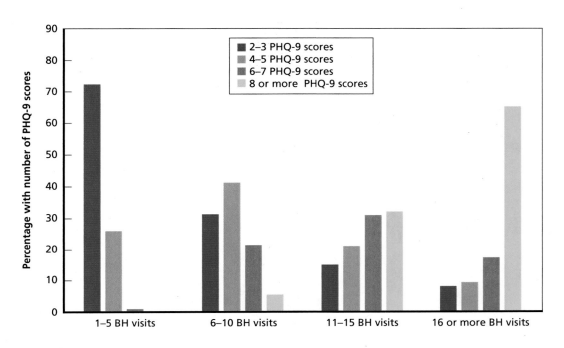

Comparison of Outcome Scores for Depression Using Army and NQF Methodologies

The measures used to track response and remission outcomes for depression are based on NQF-endorsed measures #1884, Depression Response at Six Months—Progress Towards Remission, and #0711, Depression Remission in Six Months (NQF, 2018). These measures were developed by MN Community Measurement and are used to track depression outcomes in the state of Minnesota with annually published statewide and individual clinic performance results (MN Community Measurement, 2017). In addition, in 2017, these measures were added to the HEDIS roster for the Electronic Clinical Data System (ECDS); facilities with the requisite data systems can submit HEDIS data for these measures in an automated fashion (National Committee for Quality Assurance, 2018).

We examined the implications of using the Army's methodology to compute depression outcome rates compared with the NQF methodology for depression outcomes (NQF, 2018). There are several ways that two methodologies differ, which make any comparison between Army and NQF measure results difficult. The differences are listed below and summarized in Table 3.5:

Figure 3.6
Percentage of Soldiers in the Anxiety Outcome Monitoring Sample (n = 4,282) with Specified Number of GAD-7 Scores, by Number of BH Specialty Visits in Direct Care, 2016–2017

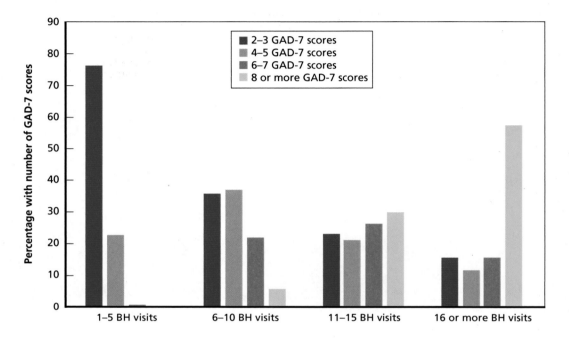

Table 3.4
Outcomes for PTSD, Depression, and Anxiety Using the Army Methodology, 2016–2017

Outcome	PTSD (n = 3,264) % (n)	Depression (n = 3,801) % (n)	Anxiety (n = 4,282) % (n)
Response	34.8 (1,137)	22.4 (851)	13.6 (584)
Remission	12.9 (420)	22.4 (850)	27.0 (1,154)
Response or remission	35.1 (1,145)	44.8 (1,701)	40.6 (1,738)

- Definition of depression: The Army uses ICD-10 major depressive disorder (MDD) codes to identify those with a diagnosis of depression. NQF uses ICD-10 codes for MDD as well as the code for dysthymia (excluding those with a diagnosis of personality disorder or bipolar disorder), resulting in the inclusion of more individuals than just those with MDD.
- Denominator selection: The Army selects individuals with an elevated initial PHQ-9 score and at least one follow-up score. The NQF selects individuals

Table 3.5
Comparison of Army and NQF Methodologies for Monitoring Depression Response and Remission

Army Criteria	NQF Criteria
Outpatient BH visit: • ICD-10 code for major depressive disorder • Code in position 1, 2, or 3	Outpatient BH visit: • ICD-10 code for major depressive disorder or dysthymia • Code in position 1 (specialty care) • No diagnosis of personality/bipolar disorder
New treatment episode (NTE): No BH care for major depressive disorder in 6 months before BH intake specialty visit	N/A
PHQ-9 score ≥10 (no missing data) +/- 30 days of NTE start date	PHQ-9 score ≥10 (no missing data) in months 1–2 of measurement period (for a 9-month measurement period)
At least one follow-up PHQ-9 score (no missing data) 1 to 6 months after the initial score	N/A
Response: 5-point reduction in last PHQ-9 score AND last score >7	Response: 50% reduction in last PHQ-9 score
Remission: 5-point reduction in last PHQ-9 score AND last score ≤7	Remission: Last PHQ-9 score <5

NOTE: Soldiers were selected from those with at least one direct care outpatient BH specialty visit between January and September 2016.

on the basis of an elevated initial PHQ-9 score alone. Those with an elevated score remain in the NQF denominator, regardless of follow-up. Those without a follow-up score are considered a "fail" according to the NQF measures. Dropping patients without a follow-up score from the denominator, as the Army methodology does, creates a higher performance rate than would be computed without those exclusions. The excluded patients include those who may not have returned to care as recommended but also those who may have improved sufficiently and are no longer in need of care. Unlike NQF, the Army also limits the sample to those with an NTE (no BH treatment for the diagnosis in the past six months). The NQF methodology does not make this restriction, making it possible to include those who may be mid-treatment but with moderate to severe symptoms.

• Follow-up period: The Army selects the last PHQ-9 score in one to six months. The NQF (as of 2017) selects the last score in five to seven months (six months plus or minus 30 days). As of 2018, the follow-up period for the NQF measure has been expanded to four to eight months (six months plus or minus 60 days). The longer NQF follow-up period may allow for a greater opportunity to capture those who reach response or remission.

- Definition of depression *response* (based on PHQ-9): The Army defines *response* as at least a five-point reduction in score and a last score greater than 7. The NQF defines *response* as a 50-percent or greater reduction in the last score compared with the initial score.
- Definition of depression *remission* (based on PHQ-9): The Army defines *remission* as at least a five-point reduction in score and a last score less than or equal to 7. The NQF defines *remission* as a last score less than 5. The Army definitions create response and remission categories that are mutually exclusive, unlike the NQF definition.

Table 3.6 shows the percentage of soldiers who met the criteria for response and remission based on the Army and NQF methodologies (for both five- to seven-month and four- to eight-month follow-up periods) based on BHDP data. The Army results are based on using the Army criteria to select the 3,801 soldiers from the 112,006 soldiers who had a BH visit between January and September 2016 (Table 2.3). The NQF results are based on using the NQF criteria to select the 3,067 soldiers from the same pool of 112,006 soldiers. However, our sample is limited to those in BH specialty care and does not include depression cases in primary care. The methodologic differences make the Army and NQF results noncomparable, but the results computed from BHDP data using the NQF methodology for five- to seven-month follow-up are very similar to the published average results from MN Community Measurement (civilian population, specialty or primary care) using 2016 statewide data, which were 13.5 percent for depression response and 8 percent for depression remission (MN Community Measurement, 2016).[1] As expected, expanding the follow-up period for depression by two months to four to eight months increases the rates of response and remission based on BHDP data and using the NQF methodology.

Table 3.6
Outcomes for Depression Response and Remission Based on BHDP Data Using the Army and NQF Methodologies, 2016–2017

Depression Outcome Measure	Army (n = 3,801) % (n)	NQF (Last score in 5–7 months) (n = 3,067) % (n)	NQF (Last score in 4–8 months) (n = 3,067) % (n)
Response	22.4 (851)	13.9 (427)	18.4 (565)
Remission	22.4 (850)	6.6 (203)	8.6 (263)
Either response or remission	44.8 (1,701)	—	—

---

[1]   The MN Community Measurement results include patients in specialty and/or primary care, and results are risk-adjusted.

Another metric that MN Measurement Community reports is the rate of having a subsequent PHQ-9 score during the follow-up period for those with an elevated initial score. In 2016, the average statewide rate of PHQ-9 follow-up (those with a PHQ-9 score during the follow-up period) in Minnesota was 32.4 percent (MN Community Measurement, 2016). Approximating this rate for the Army by looking at the number of cases dropped from inclusion for no second score, the Army rate of subsequent PHQ-9 completion was 82 percent. It must be noted that the Minnesota rate includes data from both primary care and specialty providers and is likely to be lower than the rate in specialty care alone. Still, the high Army rate of PHQ-9 follow-up likely reflects the success of the BHDP in identifying and tracking soldiers with an initial elevated PHQ-9 score over time. Specifications for quality measures that are standardized allow for greater comparability across populations. However, given the Army's use of a different methodology to compute depression outcomes, the Army depression outcome results will not be comparable to published results outside of the MHS. An alternative would be to add the NQF depression measures and analyze the relevant data on a different time cycle to accommodate the measure specifications, but at the cost of some additional administrative burden.

Summary

In this chapter, we described the patterns of outcome monitoring related to BHDP implementation and uptake and the ongoing use of the system. These findings provide information that may guide the Army's continued BHDP implementation efforts in BH specialty clinics. First, during a period of six months, we examined the length of time between the soldier's initial score and final follow-up score. Overall, there were no large, systematic gaps between soldiers' first and last scores, suggesting that those in treatment were receiving the symptom measures. Less than half of each sample had first and last symptom measures about six months apart, which represents a substantial gap between measures that could make monitoring symptom change over time difficult. Most had at least three months between their initial and last scores, but a sizable minority had little time between their initial and last scores, which could translate to a limited ability to detect any meaningful changes in scores over a brief period of time. Although it could be that soldiers completed treatment in a brief period, further findings indicated that some soldiers had BH visits after their last symptom measure score and, therefore, were not administered symptom measures when they may have been indicated.

Second, we found that the majority of soldiers received multiple symptom measures over time, with approximately half of the soldiers in the PTSD and depression samples receiving at least five symptom scores. However, fewer than half of the soldiers in the anxiety sample received this number of scores. Overall, soldiers with lengthier periods between their first and last scores had more scores recorded; this pattern was consistent across the PTSD, depression, and anxiety samples.

Third, for each sample, we examined the relationship between the number of BH specialty visits and the number of scores received. For all three samples, soldiers who received more BH care visits had more scores, and soldiers with fewer BH care specialty visits had fewer scores. Although this was generally the case across the samples, there were more soldiers in the anxiety sample who had frequent BH visits but only received a few scores (e.g., 16 percent of those with 16 or more BH visits only received two or three GAD-7 scores). Still, this series of analyses is a promising indicator that clinicians are using BHDP to track soldiers' symptoms. However, especially for the anxiety samples, there is some room for improvement: There were some lengthy gaps between first and last scores, and some soldiers who received multiple BH visits had only a few scores recorded.

In the second half of the chapter, we compared two approaches to define the response to treatment and remission outcome measures using BHDP data. First, we found that, using the Army's definition of these outcomes, rates of "response or remission" were highest for depression, followed by anxiety, and then PTSD. The rate of response alone was highest for PTSD, and the rate of remission was highest for anxiety. Next, we examined how the Army's methodology used to measure outcomes for depression differed from the NQF methodology for these outcomes. The Army and NQF definitions differed in multiple ways, such as definition of depression, denominator selection (including whether to include or exclude soldiers with no follow-up score and whether to require an NTE), length of follow-up period, and definition of score reduction. These differences make the response and remission outcomes for depression noncomparable across the two methods and make it difficult to compare findings from the Army's outcome definition with outcome results for civilian populations outside of the MHS.

CHAPTER FOUR

Characteristics and Representativeness of Soldiers in the Multivariate Analysis Samples

In this chapter, we present the demographic and service characteristics of soldiers in the PTSD, depression, and anxiety multivariate analysis samples at the time of their initial scores. We also describe outpatient utilization and comorbid diagnoses during the period between the initial and last scores and the average first and last symptom scores. Our multivariate analyses presented in Chapter Five include a subset of soldiers who were seen in Army behavioral health settings (see Chapter Two for eligibility criteria). Because of this, our analyses to identify pretreatment and treatment variables that were associated with outcomes may not generalize to all soldiers seen in Army behavioral health. To assess whether the soldiers included in our multivariate analyses were representative of other soldiers who were seen in BH specialty care at least once with these target diagnoses, we compared the characteristics of each sample with soldiers who had at least one BH visit for the target diagnosis but who *did not* meet the other sample eligibility criteria (e.g., a new treatment episode, a sufficiently elevated first symptom score, one additional symptom score in the subsequent 31 to 180 days).[1] While there are several potential comparison groups to evaluate representativeness, we identified a group that was seen in Army BH with a target diagnosis that did not meet criteria for sample inclusion. In sensitivity analyses using a comparison group that had at least two BH visits with the target diagnosis (not shown), the pattern of results were similar to what we present in this chapter. Because the focus of this chapter is on understanding the characteristics and representativeness of the soldiers included in our multivariate analyses, the analyses in this chapter use the multivariate analysis sample, which are also used in the multivariate analyses reported in Chapter Five.[2] Some key findings are the following:

---

[1] The comparison group of soldiers with at least one direct care BH specialty visit for the target condition was defined as having at least one direct care BH specialty visit with the target condition diagnosis (in position 1–3), with provider type 1 or 2, being other than a TCON or group appointment.

[2] See Table 2.5 for a description of the various samples used in the report.

- Across the PTSD, depression, and anxiety samples, most soldiers had been deployed and were male, white, non-Hispanic, and 25 to 44 years old.
- Outpatient utilization was highest among soldiers with PTSD and was lowest among those with anxiety.
- Comorbidity was similar across the PTSD, depression, and anxiety samples.
- Soldiers who were excluded from the multivariate analysis tended to be older and included more women, more officers and warrant officers, and more soldiers who had deployed.

Characteristics of PTSD, Depression, and Anxiety Multivariate Analysis Samples

Table 4.1 presents the characteristics of the three samples. About three out of four soldiers in the PTSD, depression, and anxiety samples were male (81 percent, 72 percent, and 75 percent, respectively). About half of soldiers in the PTSD, depression, and anxiety samples were white, non-Hispanic (47 percent, 44 percent, and 50 percent, respectively). A large majority of the three samples were between the ages of 25 and 44 (from 69 to 78 percent). The majority of soldiers in all three samples had been deployed since September 11, 2001.

Although these data are presented together in Table 4.1, we advise caution in directly comparing the PTSD, depression, and anxiety samples because there is considerable overlap between them. For example, 12–17 percent of each sample overlapped with one other sample, and 4–6 percent of soldiers in a given sample were also in the other two samples. With that caution, we note some observable differences in demographic and service characteristics. For example, there were proportionately more men in the PTSD sample than in the depression and anxiety samples; rates of men were comparable between the depression and anxiety samples. The anxiety sample included more white, non-Hispanic soldiers and fewer black, non-Hispanic soldiers than the PTSD or depression samples; the PTSD and depression samples had comparable rates for these two groups. The three samples had comparable proportions of soldiers identifying as Hispanic and as other race/ethnicity. In terms of age, more of those in the PTSD sample were over 35 years old than in the depression and anxiety samples. Across samples, about nine out of ten soldiers were enlisted. There was a large difference for deployment history, with a higher percentage of the PTSD sample (87 percent) having been deployed since September 11, 2001, than the depression (64 percent) or anxiety (69 percent) samples.

Table 4.2 presents data on outpatient utilization, comorbid diagnoses, and symptom scores for the three samples for the period between the initial and last scores. The data capture outpatient utilization associated with any diagnosis (i.e., medical or BH) and with a primary BH diagnosis, including both direct and purchased care visits.

Table 4.1
Demographic and Service Characteristics of PTSD,
Depression, and Anxiety Multivariate Analysis Samples,
2016–2017

Characteristic	PTSD % (n)	Depression % (n)	Anxiety % (n)
Total	100.0 (1,528)	100.0 (1,849)	100.0 (2,592)
Sex			
Female	18.6 (284)	28.2 (521)	24.9 (646)
Male	81.4 (1,244)	71.8 (1,328)	75.1 (1,946)
Race/ethnicity			
White, non-Hispanic	47.0 (718)	44.2 (817)	50.4 (1,307)
Black, non-Hispanic	30.2 (461)	32.3 (597)	28.2 (730)
Hispanic	15.4 (236)	16.3 (301)	14.8 (383)
Other/unknown	7.4 (113)	7.2 (134)	6.6 (172)
Age			
18–24	13.5 (206)	23.9 (441)	22.5 (584)
25–34	39.1 (598)	39.0 (721)	39.6 (1,026)
35–44	38.4 (587)	30.0 (555)	31.8 (825)
45 and over	9.0 (137)	7.1 (132)	6.1 (157)
Pay grade			
Enlisted (E1–E9)	89.3 (1,364)	89.7 (1,658)	89.8 (2,327)
Officer/warrant officer (O1–O6, warrant)	10.7 (164)	10.3 (191)	10.2 (265)
Deployment history			
Not deployed since 9/11/2001	13.0 (424)	35.6 (1,352)	30.8 (1,320)
Deployed since 9/11/2001	87.0 (2,840)	64.4 (2,449)	69.2 (2,962)

NOTES: Characteristics were assessed at the time of the initial score. There is overlap of soldiers included across the three samples, so the reader should use caution when making direct comparisons (see Figure 2.2).

Table 4.2
Outpatient Visits and Comorbidity During Follow-Up and Symptom Severity of PTSD, Depression, and Anxiety Multivariate Analysis Samples, 2016–2017

Characteristic	PTSD (n = 1,528)	Depression (n = 1,849)	Anxiety (n = 2,592)
Number of outpatient visits, any diagnosis, median[a]	34	32	26
Number of outpatient visits with any primary BH diagnosis, median[a]	16	15	11
Comorbidities, % (n)[a]			
Adjustment disorders	45.9 (702)	50.4 (931)	49.0 (1,271)
Alcohol abuse/dependence	16.6 (253)	16.5 (306)	12.3 (318)
Anxiety[b]	47.6 (728)	47.0 (869)	97.4 (2,525)
Depression[b]	52.6 (804)	98.5 (1,822)	48.1 (1,246)
Drug abuse/dependence	2.9 (44)	3.4 (62)	2.9 (74)
PTSD[b]	99.1 (1,514)	43.0 (795)	40.3 (1,044)
Sleep disorders/symptoms	67.9 (1,037)	62.8 (1,161)	62.5 (1,619)
Target condition symptom severity (PCL-5, PHQ-9, GAD-7)			
Initial score, mean (SD)	50.1 (13.0)	17.8 (4.5)	15.4 (3.5)
Last score, mean (SD)	45.5 (18.5)	13.8 (6.9)	12.2 (6.2)

[a] Includes direct and purchased care visits from initial elevated symptom score to last score.

[b] Small discrepancies between target diagnoses within the samples (e.g., 99 percent of PTSD sample had PTSD) reflect the timing of diagnosis relative to the initial elevated score, as some soldiers received the target diagnosis prior to the first elevated score.

NOTES: SD = standard deviation. There is overlap of soldiers included across the three samples, so the reader should use caution when making direct comparisons (see Figure 2.2).

Soldiers in the PTSD sample had the most outpatient visits (for any reason and for a BH primary diagnosis), while soldiers in the anxiety sample had the fewest outpatient visits.

With the exception of the sample diagnoses, comorbidity was generally the same across the samples. About half of the PTSD, depression, and anxiety samples each had comorbid adjustment disorders. There was quite a bit of overlap between the other two targeted diagnoses in each sample: About half of the PTSD and anxiety samples had depression, and about 40 percent in the depression and anxiety samples had PTSD. Most of the soldiers in each sample (63–68 percent) had comorbid sleep disorders or symptoms. The anxiety sample had a slightly lower rate of a comorbid alcohol abuse or dependence diagnosis (13 percent) than the PTSD (17 percent) and depression (17 percent) samples. About 3 percent of each sample had a comorbid diagnosis of drug abuse or dependence.

Mean scores on the symptom measures declined from the initial score to last score, with a change from average first score to average last score of −4.6, −4.0, and −3.2 points for the PCL-5, PHQ-9, and GAD-7, respectively. However, even at last follow-up, as a whole, the scores still crested above a clinically meaningful severity level (mean score of 45 on the PCL-5, mean score of 14 on the PHQ-9, and mean score of 12 on the GAD-7). These average scores were not case-adjusted, but the means suggest that, at the group level, there was not a clinically significant amount of change. None of the average score reductions met the Army-defined threshold of a clinically significant decrease in score (ten points for the PCL-5 and five points for the PHQ-9 and GAD-7). Studies of the PCL suggest a five-point reduction as a minimum threshold for determining whether an individual has responded to treatment and ten points as a minimum threshold for determining whether the improvement is clinically meaningful (Weathers et al., 2013).[3] Studies of the PHQ-9 suggest a score reduction of five points as a clinically significant change for depression (Löwe et al., 2004).

Representativeness of the PTSD, Depression, and Anxiety Multivariate Analysis Samples

To assess whether soldiers in the PTSD multivariate analysis sample were representative of other soldiers with PTSD excluded from the sample, we compared the characteristics of soldiers in the PTSD multivariate analysis sample with soldiers with at least one BH visit for PTSD who did not meet the other sample eligibility criteria

---

[3]   This is based on the PCL and is assumed as a reasonable range for the PCL-5 while further studies of the PCL-5 are conducted.

(see Table 4.3).[4] Although there were no statistically significant differences in gender and race/ethnicity between the two groups, there were significant differences in age, pay grade, and deployment history. Soldiers in the PTSD multivariate analysis sample were younger and included a somewhat larger proportion of soldiers with no history of deployments than those excluded from the sample (13 percent versus 9 percent). While this result may seem counter to what might be expected, it reflects that PTSD also occurs in nondeployed service members. PTSD in garrison could result from a variety of traumatic events, including sexual assault, automobile accidents, and training accidents. Less is known about the prevalence of PTSD in the nondeployed, but one survey of veterans from the Operation Enduring Freedom and Operation Iraqi Freedom (OEF/OIF) era revealed an overall weighted prevalence of a positive screen for PTSD of 15.8 percent among OEF/OIF veterans and 10.9 percent in nondeployed veterans (Dursa et al., 2014). It is possible that soldiers who had a history of deployment were less likely to continue in care, making them less likely to be in our sample (e.g., less likely to have a follow-up score or follow-up visit).

When examining the representativeness of the depression multivariate analysis sample, we found statistically significant differences between the depression sample and the comparison group on all of the variables we examined (see Table 4.4). The depression sample included more men and fewer white, non-Hispanic soldiers; these soldiers were also younger, more likely to be enlisted, and less likely to have been deployed than those excluded from the sample.

When examining the representativeness of the anxiety multivariate analysis sample, we found statistically significant differences between the depression sample and the comparison group on all variables included in our analysis (see Table 4.5). Soldiers in the anxiety multivariate analysis sample were less likely to be male and white, non-Hispanic; they were less likely to have a history of deployment and more likely to be younger, enlisted personnel than those excluded from the sample.

Summary

There were few notable differences across soldiers in the PTSD, depression, and anxiety multivariate analysis samples. This would be expected, given the overlap between these samples and the comorbidity typically seen among these diagnoses. Across our samples, most soldiers were male, and about half were white, non-Hispanic. Most were between 25 and 44 years old and had been deployed since September 11, 2001.

Given the overlap, direct comparisons of the samples can be challenging, but we observed some differences. For example, the PTSD sample included more men

---

[4]   The comparison group of soldiers with at least one direct care BH specialty visit for the target condition was defined as having at least one direct care BH specialty visit with the target condition diagnosis (in position 1–3), with provider type 1 or 2, being other than a TCON or group appointment.

Table 4.3
Demographic Characteristics of PTSD Multivariate Analysis Sample and Those with One or More BH Visits Who Were Excluded from the PTSD Sample, 2016–2017

Characteristic	PTSD Multivariate Analysis Sample[a] (n = 1,528), % (n)	At Least One BH Visit for PTSD but Excluded from PTSD Sample[b] (n = 9,558), % (n)	P-Value
Gender			
Female	18.6 (284)	17.2 (1,648)	0.1984
Male	81.4 (1,244)	82.8 (7,910)	
Race/ethnicity			
White, non-Hispanic	47.0 (718)	48.3 (4,614)	0.5305
Black, non-Hispanic	30.2 (461)	29.9 (2,853)	
Hispanic	15.4 (236)	14.2 (1,353)	
Other/unknown	7.4 (113)	7.7 (738)	
Age			
18–24	13.5 (206)	8.7 (827)	<0.0001
25–34	39.1 (598)	34.6 (3,304)	
35–44	38.4 (587)	43.4 (4,148)	
45 and over	9.0 (137)	13.4 (1,279)	
Pay grade			
Enlisted (E1–E9)	89.3 (1,364)	85.1 (8,136)	<0.0001
Officer/warrant officer (O1–O6, warrant)	10.7 (164)	14.9 (1,420)	
Deployment history			
Not deployed since 9/11/2001	13.0 (424)	9.2 (907)	<0.0001
Deployed since 9/11/2001	87.0 (2,840)	90.8 (8,975)	

[a] For the multivariate analysis sample, the characteristics were measured at the time of the initial elevated *score*.

[b] Based on the PTSD sample selection criteria described in Chapter Two. The characteristics were measured at the time of the initial *visit* for this comparison group.

Table 4.4
Demographic Characteristics of Depression Multivariate Analysis Sample and Those with One or More BH Visits Who Were Excluded from the Depression Sample, 2016–2017

Characteristic	Depression Multivariate Analysis Sample[a] (n = 1,849), % (n)	At Least One BH Visit for Depression but Excluded from Depression Sample[b] (n = 7,924), % (n)	P-Value
Gender			
Female	28.2 (521)	31.1 (2,466)	0.0134
Male	71.8 (1,328)	68.9 (5,458)	
Race/ethnicity			
White, non-Hispanic	44.2 (817)	49.9 (3,956)	<0.0001
Black, non-Hispanic	32.3 (597)	29.4 (2,328)	
Hispanic	16.3 (301)	13.5 (1,068)	
Other/unknown	7.2 (134)	7.2 (572)	
Age			
15–24	23.9 (441)	22.9 (1,814)	0.0199
25–34	39.0 (721)	36.8 (2,917)	
35–44	30.0 (555)	31.2 (2,471)	
45 and over	7.1 (132)	9.1 (722)	
Pay grade			
Enlisted (E1–E9)	89.7 (1,658)	85.1 (6,735)	<0.0001
Officer/warrant officer (O1–O6, warrant)	10.3 (191)	14.9 (1,179)	
Deployment history			
Not deployed since 9/11/2001	35.6 (1,352)	31.8 (2,574)	<0.0001
Deployed since 9/11/2001	64.4 (2,449)	68.2 (5,531)	

[a] The characteristics were measured at the time of the initial elevated *score* for the multivariate analysis sample.

[b] Based on the depression sample selection criteria described in Chapter Two. The characteristics were measured at the time of the initial *visit* for this comparison group.

Table 4.5
Demographic Characteristics of Anxiety Multivariate Analysis Sample and Those with One or More BH Visits Who Were Excluded from the Anxiety Sample, 2016–2017

Characteristic	Anxiety Multivariate Analysis Sample[a] (n = 2,592), % (n)	At Least One BH Visit for Anxiety but Excluded from Anxiety Sample[b] (n = 13,752), % (n)	P-Value
Gender			
Female	24.9 (646)	23.1 (3,171)	0.0396
Male	75.1 (1,946)	76.9 (10,581)	
Race/ethnicity			
White, non-Hispanic	50.4 (1,307)	57.0 (7,840)	<0.0001
Black, non-Hispanic	28.2 (730)	23.7 (3,253)	
Hispanic	14.8 (383)	12.9 (1,770)	
Other/unknown	6.6 (172)	6.5 (889)	
Age			
15–24	22.5 (584)	21.0 (2,888)	0.0006
25–34	39.6 (1,026)	39.3 (5,397)	
35–44	31.8 (825)	31.4 (4,316)	
45 and over	6.1 (157)	8.4 (1,151)	
Pay grade			
Enlisted (E1–E9)	89.8 (2,327)	85.7 (11,774)	<0.0001
Officer/warrant officer (O1–O6, warrant)	10.2 (265)	14.3 (1,964)	
Deployment history			
Not deployed since 9/11/2001	30.8 (1,320)	28.0 (3,885)	0.0003
Deployed since 9/11/2001	69.2 (2,962)	72.0 (9,990)	

[a] The characteristics were measured at the time of the initial *score* for the multivariate analysis sample.

[b] Based on the anxiety sample selection criteria described in Chapter Two. The characteristics were measured at the time of the initial *visit* for this comparison group.

than the depression and anxiety samples. The anxiety sample was made up of more white, non-Hispanic soldiers and fewer black, non-Hispanic soldiers than the PTSD or depression samples. The PTSD sample was also older and included more soldiers with a history of deployment than the depression and anxiety samples. The PTSD sample had more outpatient health care utilization for both BH and non-BH diagnoses than the other two samples. Comorbidity was similar across the samples, with about half or slightly less than half of each sample having a diagnosis of one of the other target diagnoses (e.g., 54 percent of the PTSD sample had comorbid depression, and 49 percent had comorbid anxiety). There were similarities in rates of other comorbid diagnoses as well, such as sleep disorders or symptoms, adjustment disorders, and drug abuse or dependence, although the anxiety sample had a slightly lower rate of comorbid alcohol abuse or dependence than the other two samples. Mean symptom scores declined between the initial and follow-up score, but the magnitude of change was small across the measures (3.2–4.6 points).

There were significant differences between the PTSD, depression, and anxiety multivariate analysis samples and a comparison group of soldiers who had received at least one BH visit for the target diagnosis but who did not meet the other sample eligibility criteria of a new treatment episode, a sufficiently elevated first symptom score, and at least one additional symptom score in the subsequent 31 to 180 days. Soldiers who were excluded tended to be older; this group also included a greater proportion of women and officers or warrant officers, as well as soldiers who had deployed. It is possible that soldiers who had a history of deployment were less likely to continue in care, making them less likely to be in our sample (e.g., less likely to have a follow-up score or follow-up visit). These differences were seen across diagnoses. In addition, soldiers excluded from the anxiety multivariate analysis sample were more likely to be white, non-Hispanic. Given these differences, we advise caution in generalizing the results from our analyses to a broader group of soldiers with the target diagnoses.

CHAPTER FIVE

Identifying Pretreatment and Treatment Predictors of PTSD, Depression, and Anxiety Outcomes

In this chapter, we describe the analyses conducted to identify pretreatment and treatment factors that are associated with improved clinical outcomes in soldiers in BH specialty care for the target diagnoses (i.e., PTSD, depression, and anxiety disorders). Analyses in this chapter use the multivariate analysis sample (see Chapter Two). Based on our analyses, key findings in this chapter include the following:

- In general, worse BH symptom severity was associated with worse outcomes, although this was less consistent for soldiers in the depression sample.
- No pretreatment factors (i.e., demographic or risk characteristics) were consistently associated with outcomes.
- Improved soldier-reported therapeutic alliance with providers was associated with better PTSD, depression, and anxiety outcomes.
- Soldiers with a greater than 30-day supply of benzodiazepine medication had poorer PTSD, depression, and anxiety outcomes.

Overview of Process for Identifying Predictors

Identifying Pretreatment Predictors

As described in Chapter Two, we used a multistep variable selection process to first identify patient pretreatment variables (i.e., risk and demographic factors; steps 1–4). We examined 57 variables representing pretreatment characteristics (including soldier demographics, military service characteristics, baseline and historical clinical characteristics, comorbid conditions, and treatment history). Full model results for these pretreatment variables are included in Appendix B (Tables B.1, B.2, and B.3 for PTSD, depression, and anxiety, respectively). Table 5.1 shows the pretreatment variables that we retained; these include pretreatment variables retained regardless of significance (e.g., age, sex) and variables that were significant for each sample. The analyses discussed in this chapter focused on the pretreatment variables that we identified in prior analyses, as well as treatment variables.

Table 5.1
Pretreatment Variables Included in the Models

Variable Type	Variable Label
Demographic data (at the time of initial score):	Marital status
	Sex
	Age
	Race/ethnicity
Service-related characteristics (at the time of initial score):	Pay grade
	Total deployments
Symptoms (30 days prior to 1 week after initial score):	General distress (BASIS score)
	Suicide risk (C-SSRS, current score)
	Alcohol consumption (AUDIT-C score)
	Function, personal/social (WRAIR PSF score)
	Function, occupational (WRAIR OF score)
	Pain, current
	Initial elevated symptom score (PCL-5, PHQ-9, or GAD-7 related to diagnostic sample and +/–30 days of the intake visit)
	Symptom score (PCL-5 for depression or anxiety sample; PHQ-9 for PTSD or anxiety sample; GAD-7 for PTSD or depression sample)
Past history (>1 month to 1 year prior to initial score):	PTSD, past history
	Depression, past history
	Anxiety, past history
	Sleep disorder/symptoms, past history
Current diagnosis (1 month prior to 1 week after initial score):	PTSD, current (for depression or anxiety sample)
	Depression, current (for PTSD or anxiety sample)
	Anxiety, current (for PTSD or depression sample)
	Sleep disorder/symptoms, current
Current psychotropic medication (in 1 month prior to initial score):	Psychotropic medication, current
Past health care utilization (>1 month to 1 year prior to initial score):	Non-MH outpatient visits
	MH outpatient visits

NOTES: C-SSRS = Columbia Suicide Severity Rating Scale; OF = occupational function.

Identifying Treatment Predictors

We examined 84 treatment predictors assessing a variety of aspects of treatment, including psychotherapy visits, individual therapy visits, group therapy visits, provider (e.g., type of provider, soldier-provider therapeutic alliance), number of E&M visits, number of BH visits, and medications dispensed (e.g., antidepressants, benzodiazepines; see Appendix A).

We included two time-related covariates in these models, such as whether the initial score was measured after the initial (intake) visit and the number of days from the initial score to the last score. Thus, the models presented in this chapter represent the final analytic models of pretreatment (demographic, risk) and treatment factors (step 9, as described in Chapter Two). Appendix B contains the estimates, confidence intervals (CIs), and p-values for all predictors in the final models for the PCL-5, PHQ-9, and GAD-7 symptom score-change continuous outcome, as well as response to treatment and remission (dichotomous) outcomes for each of the three samples. Several of the variables listed in Appendix A were evaluated and were not included in the final models (e.g., variables capturing type of provider), as outlined in multistep process described in Chapter Two.

Pretreatment and Treatment Factors Associated with Soldier Outcomes

Patient Pretreatment and Treatment Predictors of PTSD Symptom Outcomes
Pretreatment and Treatment Predictors of Continuous PTSD Symptom Change
Full model results are provided in Table B.4 in Appendix B. Table 5.2 presents the multivariate findings examining which predictors were associated with differences between the last and initial PCL-5 score for soldiers in the PTSD sample. The "Estimate" column indicates the regression coefficient, which reflects the size and direction of the relationship between the predictor and the outcome. For example, an estimate of −0.5 for the initial PCL-5 score indicates that a soldier with an initial score of 40 would expect to have a decrease in their symptom score of 20 points (i.e., −0.5 multiplied by 40) from their initial PCL-5 to the last PCL-5. As another example, the general distress score had a positive regression coefficient of 5.13, so a one-point increase in the distress score would be associated with a 5.13-point increase in the PCL-5 score from the initial PCL-5 to the last PCL-5. Seven pretreatment and five treatment factors were significantly associated with PCL-5 score changes.

In terms of pretreatment variables, greater alcohol use, PTSD symptoms, suicide risk, and depression symptoms were all significantly associated with reductions in PTSD symptoms. Greater general distress and poorer personal/social functioning were associated with a poorer PTSD outcome. Having more days between the first and last PCL score also was associated with a poorer PTSD outcome. This latter finding is not

Table 5.2
Pretreatment and Treatment Predictors of Difference Between Last and Initial PCL-5 Scores Among Soldiers in the PTSD Multivariate Analysis Sample (n = 1,528), 2016–2017

Variable	Continuous PTSD (PCL-5) Outcome	
	Estimate [CI]	P-Value
Time covariates:		
Initial score is after index visit	0.02 [–1.99, 2.03]	0.99
Total days between first-last scores	0.05 [0.02, 0.07]	0.00
Pretreatment		
Marital status		
Marital status: Divorced, separated, widowed	1.59 [–2.10, 5.28]	0.40
Marital status: Married	0.31 [–2.58, 3.20]	0.83
Marital status: Never married [reference group]		
Sex		
Female	–0.61 [–2.94, 1.72]	0.61
Age		
18–24	0.52 [–3.88, 4.92]	0.82
25–34	1.08 [–2.21, 4.37]	0.52
35–44	1.88 [–1.13, 4.89]	0.22
45–64 [reference group]		
Race/ethnicity		
Black, non-Hispanic	1.29 [–0.67, 3.25]	0.20
Hispanic	2.32 [–0.07, 4.70]	0.06
Other	0.96 [–2.27, 4.19]	0.56
White, non-Hispanic [reference group]		
Pay grade		
E1–E4	–1.02 [-4.61, 2.57]	0.58
E5–E6	0.13 [–2.71, 2.96]	0.93
E7–E9	–0.24 [–3.3, 2.83]	0.88
Officer/warrant officer [reference group]		

Table 5.2—continued

Variable	Continuous PTSD (PCL-5) Outcome	
	Estimate [CI]	P-Value
Total deployments	−0.09 [−0.71, 0.53]	0.77
General distress (BASIS score)	5.13 [2.46, 7.80]	0.00
Suicide risk (C-SSRS, current score)	−1.52 [−2.25, −0.78]	0.00
Alcohol consumption (AUDIT-C score)	−0.39 [−0.68, −0.10]	0.01
Function, personal/social (WRAIR PSF score)	0.38 [0.06, 0.69]	0.02
Initial PCL-5 score	−0.50 [−0.59, −0.41]	0.00
PHQ-9 score	−0.30 [−0.56, −0.04]	0.02
Treatment		
Therapeutic Alliance Questionnaire score	−0.37 [−0.49, −0.25]	0.00
Group therapy visits, direct care, primary diagnosis, per month		
>0–<3 visits	3.04 [0.84, 5.24]	0.01
3–4 visits	5.56 [−5.63, 16.74]	0.33
>4 visits	−5.22 [−14.97, 4.53]	0.29
No visits [reference group]		
BH visits, direct care, without IOP, primary diagnosis, per month	1.00 [0.41, 1.58]	0.00
Benzodiazepine, days' supply		
0 days [reference group]		
1–30 days	2.09 [−0.69, 4.88]	0.14
>30 days	4.24 [1.59, 6.89]	0.00
SSRI/SNRI/antidepressant and psychotherapy	1.84 [0.04, 3.63]	0.04

NOTES: Current = 30 days prior to 1 week after initial symptom score.
IOP = intensive outpatient program; SNRI = serotonin-norepinephrine reuptake inhibitor; SSRI = selective serotonin reuptake inhibitor.

surprising, given that those with more severe PTSD would likely be receiving more treatment sessions over time.

In terms of treatment variables, only one of the five statistically significant variables was associated with improved symptoms. Stronger therapeutic alliance between the soldier and his or her provider (as reported by the soldier) was associated with a decrease in PTSD symptoms. The other four significant variables were associated with a worse PTSD outcome: frequency of group therapy for PTSD, receipt of benzodiazepines, receipt of both antidepressant medication and psychotherapy, and number of direct care BH visits for PTSD. These results suggest that more group therapy sessions for PTSD, having more than a 30-day supply of benzodiazepines, receiving both antidepressant medication and at least one PTSD-related psychotherapy session after intake, and more frequent BH visits for PTSD were associated with a poorer PTSD outcome for soldiers.

Pretreatment and Treatment Predictors of Response to Treatment for Soldiers with PTSD

Response to treatment is a dichotomous variable, defined by the Army methodology as a ten-point or greater reduction in PCL-5 score from the initial to the last score. The pattern of results for response to treatment was nearly identical to those for the continuous PTSD symptom change outcome. Full model results are provided in Table B.4 in Appendix B. In terms of pretreatment variables, more severe PTSD symptoms and greater suicide risk were associated with a higher likelihood of a PTSD treatment response; both were observed for the continuous PTSD outcome in the full model. However, the findings for alcohol consumption and depression severity observed for the continuous PTSD outcome were not replicated, such that alcohol consumption and depression scores were not significantly associated with response to treatment as they were for the continuous change score outcome. However, as observed for the continuous PTSD outcome, more general distress and poorer personal/social functioning were associated with lower likelihood of response to treatment. Having more days between the first and last scores was also associated with a lower likelihood of response and with a poorer PTSD outcome, as it was in the continuous model.

Regarding treatment factors, three of the five significant findings observed for the continuous change score outcomes were replicated by the response to treatment findings. Therapeutic alliance again emerged as the sole treatment factor that was associated with better PTSD outcomes, such that a better working relationship between the soldier and his or her provider (as reported by the soldier) was associated with a higher likely of a treatment response. As with the continuous outcome findings, greater than zero but less than three direct care group therapy sessions per month for PTSD as the primary diagnosis (compared with zero sessions) and more than a 30-day supply of benzodiazepines were associated with a lower likelihood of a PTSD treatment response for soldiers. The findings observed for receipt of antidepressant medication and psychotherapy, as well as the number of direct care BH visits for PTSD without any intensive outpatient care per month, were not replicated, as there were no significant findings observed for response to treatment.

Pretreatment and Treatment Predictors of Remission for Soldiers with PTSD

Remission is a dichotomous variable defined by the Army methodology as a final follow-up PCL-5 score of 22 or less. Full model results are provided in Table B.4 in Appendix B. Three of the significant findings for the pretreatment predictors observed for the continuous outcome of PTSD change scores were replicated by the findings for remission: A higher level of alcohol use was associated with an increased likelihood of remission, poorer personal/social functioning was associated with a lower likelihood of remission, and greater general distress was associated with a lower likelihood of remission. The findings for poorer personal/social functioning and greater general distress were also replicated for the response outcome. Contrary to both the change scores and response to treatment outcomes, higher initial PTSD severity scores were associated with a *lower* likelihood of PTSD remission at final follow-up.

Therapeutic alliance was associated with better PTSD outcomes, such that a stronger therapeutic alliance was associated with an increased likelihood of remission. This finding was replicated by both the continuous change score outcome and the response to treatment outcome. Finally, a larger number of direct care BH visits for PTSD as the primary diagnosis without any intensive outpatient care per month was associated with a lower likelihood of remission. This finding was a replication of the finding for the continuous change score outcome.

Summary of Models to Predict PTSD Symptom Outcomes

The final multivariate models suggested that, for pretreatment factors, more reports of such BH symptoms as frequent alcohol use, suicide risk, and more severe PTSD were associated with better PTSD outcomes over time, while greater general distress and poorer functioning were associated with worse PTSD outcomes over time. It is possible that soldiers who were more severe in several BH areas may have seen reductions in PTSD symptoms because those who are more severe have more room for improvement during treatment. The identified BH symptoms of heavy alcohol use, depression, and suicidality have much overlap with PTSD symptoms, and improvements in PTSD symptoms likely would also lead to reductions in the other symptoms. It should be noted that the treatment soldiers received may not have been specific to PTSD, and it was likely that the other BH symptoms of heavy alcohol use, depression, and suicidality were addressed during treatment. As those targeted symptoms reduced, it is possible that PTSD symptoms also reduced. For example, a soldier who was drinking heavily to cope with PTSD symptoms may have been treated for both PTSD and heavy alcohol use. As the soldier learned to cope better with PTSD symptoms without the heavy use of alcohol, the PTSD symptoms likely abated. Such reductions in co-occurring symptoms have been documented in clinical trials of military populations in treatment settings (Norman et al., 2010; van Minnen et al., 2015).

Findings related to pretreatment factors were similar across the three PTSD outcomes. One exception was the direction of the effect for the initial PCL-5 score, which indicated that more severe PTSD symptoms at treatment start were associated with greater reductions in PTSD symptoms over time and an increased likelihood of a response to treatment, but with lower likelihood of remission. That is, soldiers with a higher initial PCL-5 score had a higher likelihood of improvement in their PTSD symptoms (continuous outcome and response to treatment), which is not uncommon in observational analyses because individuals with higher initial scores have more opportunity for a score decrease, compared with individuals whose initial score is low. However, the finding for PTSD remission was not consistent with the direction of the PCL-5 score change outcome or the PTSD response outcome. That is, initial PCL-5 scores were associated with a lower likelihood that soldiers would achieve remission, suggesting an inconsistency in the findings across the three outcomes.

One treatment factor finding that was significantly associated with all three PTSD outcomes and in the same direction was therapeutic alliance, such that a higher score on the soldier-reported therapeutic alliance between the soldier and his or her provider was associated with better PTSD outcomes. Much research on the therapeutic relationship between patient and provider in BH care settings supports this finding. Positive patient perceptions of their relationships with providers appear to be an essential component of treating PTSD among soldiers. This factor emerged as the only treatment factor that was associated with better PTSD outcomes. The therapeutic alliance score used in this study is computed from the DoD/VA-developed Therapeutic Alliance Questionnaire. It is based on three items reported by the patient (on a scale of 0–10 each, 10 being best) addressing the provider-patient working relationship, the mutuality of agreed-upon goals, and the level of agreement on the best approach to the patient's problems. DoD and VA have done some work to understand the psychometric properties of the measure, but this has not yet been published. It is not known how this measure of alliance relates to the Working Alliance Inventory (WAI; Hatcher and Gillaspy, 2006), and, as yet, there are still no recommended cutoffs or interpretation for the score. Other significant treatment factor findings suggested that more treatment—such as more frequent BH care visits, a combination of antianxiety/antidepressant medication and psychotherapy, and larger dispensed supplies of benzodiazepine medication—was associated with poorer PTSD outcomes. A logical reason for such findings is that soldiers who were more severe received more care, including BH care visits and prescribed medications.

Pretreatment and Treatment Predictors of Depression Symptom Outcomes
Pretreatment and Treatment Predictors of Continuous Depression Symptom Change

Table 5.3 presents the multivariate findings examining factors that were associated with differences between the last follow-up PHQ-9 score and the initial PHQ-9 score for soldiers receiving BH specialty care in the depression sample. Full model results are provided in Table B.5 in Appendix B. The "Estimate" column indicates the size

Table 5.3
Pretreatment and Treatment Predictors of Difference Between Last and Initial PHQ-9 Scores Among Soldiers in the Depression Multivariate Analysis Sample (n = 1,849), 2016–2017

Variable	Continuous Depression (PHQ-9) Outcome	
	Estimate [CI]	P-Value
Time covariates:		
Initial score is after index visit	0.27 [−0.49, 1.03]	0.49
Total days between first-last scores	0.02 [0.02, 0.03]	0.00
Pretreatment		
Marital status		
Divorced, separated, widowed	1.76 [0.63, 2.89]	0.00
Married	1.27 [0.47, 2.06]	0.00
Never married [reference group]		
Sex		
Female	−0.41 [−1.07, 0.24]	0.21
Age		
18–24	0.13 [−1.36, 1.62]	0.86
25–34	0.19 [−1.03, 1.40]	0.76
35–44	0.25 [−0.89, 1.38]	0.67
45–64 [reference group]		
Race/ethnicity		
Black, non-Hispanic	0.24 [−0.43, 0.90]	0.48
Hispanic	0.73 [−0.07, 1.52]	0.07
Other	0.35 [−0.75, 1.44]	0.54
White, non-Hispanic [reference group]		
Pay grade		
E1–E4	−0.11 [−1.31, 1.09]	0.86
E5–E6	0.26 [−0.73, 1.25]	0.61
E7–E9	−0.23 [−1.32, 0.86]	0.68
Officer/warrant officer [reference group]		
Total deployments	0.01 [−0.21, 0.24]	0.92

Table 5.3—continued

Variable	Continuous Depression (PHQ-9) Outcome	
	Estimate [CI]	P-Value
Suicide risk (C-SSRS, current score)	−0.37 [−0.56, −0.17]	0.00
Function, personal/social (WRAIR PSF score)	0.23 [0.13, 0.32]	0.00
Pain, current	1.01 [0.41, 1.61]	0.00
Initial PHQ-9 score	−0.79 [−0.87, −0.71]	0.00
PCL-5 score	0.08 [0.06, 0.10]	0.00
Sleep disorder/symptoms, past history	1.33 [0.75, 1.92]	0.00
Treatment		
Therapeutic Alliance Questionnaire score	−0.19 [−0.23, −0.15]	0.00
Individual therapy visits, all care, any MH, per month		
0–<2 visits	−1.52 [−2.46, −0.57]	0.00
2–4 visits	−0.98 [−1.89, −0.07]	0.03
>4 [reference group]		
BH visits, direct care, with IOP, primary/secondary diagnosis, per month	0.10 [−0.07, 0.28]	0.25
BH visits, direct care, without IOP, primary diagnosis, per month	−0.14 [−0.41, 0.13]	0.31
Benzodiazepine, days' supply		
0 days [reference group]		
1–30 days	0.96 [−0.11, 2.02]	0.08
>30 days	0.96 [0.04, 1.88]	0.04

NOTE: Current = 30 days prior to 1 week after initial symptom score; past history = 1 year to 30 days prior to initial symptom score.

and direction of the relationship between the predictor and the outcome. Specifically, a negative number suggests that the predictor was associated with a decreased PHQ-9 score between the initial and last scores, while a positive estimate suggests that the predictor will be associated with an increase in the change in PHQ-9 between the initial and last score. Nine pretreatment and four treatment factors emerged as significant predictors of PHQ-9 score changes.

In terms of pretreatment variables, only two factors were associated with a better depression outcome: PTSD symptoms and suicide risk. Seven other pretreatment variables were associated with a poorer depression outcome: a past history of poor sleep; poorer personal and social functioning; PTSD severity; current pain; a greater number of days between the first and last PHQ-9 score; being divorced, separated, or widowed (as compared with never having been married); and currently being married (as compared with never having been married).

Three treatment factors were associated with decreased depression symptom scores. Compared with receiving individual therapy (for any MH diagnosis) more than four times per month, receiving one or fewer or between two and four individual therapy sessions per month was associated with reduced depression symptoms. Stronger therapeutic alliance between the soldier and his or her provider was also associated with better depression outcomes. One treatment factor was associated with poorer depression outcomes: more than a 30-day supply of benzodiazepines (as compared with no supply).

Pretreatment and Treatment Predictors of Response to Treatment for Soldiers with Depression

Response to treatment was defined by a reduction of five or more points in PHQ-9 scores from the initial to last follow-up score and a final score of 8 or higher. Full model results are provided in Table B.5 in Appendix B. For pretreatment variables, similar to the continuous outcome findings for depression change scores, a more severe initial depression score was associated with an increased likelihood of a response to treatment, while poorer personal and social functioning was associated with a lower likelihood of response.

For treatment factors, as with the depression change scores outcome, therapeutic alliance again was associated with better depression outcomes, such that a better working relationship between the soldier and his or her provider (as reported by the soldier) was associated with a higher likelihood of a depression treatment response. We observed a finding not replicated in the depression change score outcome: More BH care visits for depression (primary or secondary diagnosis) per month, including IOP visits, was associated with a lower likelihood of a depression treatment response. This was not surprising given that soldiers who were more severe and failed to obtain a treatment response received more care over time.

Pretreatment and Treatment Predictors of Remission for Soldiers with Depression

Remission was defined by a reduction of five or more points in PHQ-9 scores from the initial to the last follow-up and a final follow-up score of 7 or less. Full model results are provided in Table B.5 in Appendix B. Several findings observed for the continuous change score outcome were replicated. A past history of poor sleep, poorer personal and social functioning, higher PTSD severity, current pain, and a greater number of days between the first and last PHQ-9 scores were associated with a lower likelihood of remission at follow-up. As with the continuous score change outcomes, more severe suicide risk was associated with a greater likelihood of remission at follow-up. The finding for poorer personal and social functioning was also replicated for the depression response outcome.

Two treatment factors were associated with a greater likelihood of remission. Compared with receipt of individual therapy (for any mental health diagnosis) more than four times per month, receiving one or less than one individual therapy sessions per month was associated with a greater likelihood of remission. This finding was replicated in the continuous analyses of the depression change scores. Higher therapeutic alliance was associated with better depression outcomes, such that a better therapeutic alliance was associated with a greater likelihood of depression remission. The therapeutic alliance finding was replicated for both the continuous score change and depression response outcomes.

Summary of Models to Predict Depression Symptom Outcomes

The final multivariate model's findings were somewhat mixed regarding whether greater reports of BH symptoms and poorer functioning were associated with better or worse depression outcomes. Higher initial PHQ-9 scores and greater reported suicide risk were associated with better depression outcomes over time, while poorer personal and social functioning, past history of sleep disorder or symptoms, PTSD symptoms, and pain were associated with poorer depression outcomes. These findings were generally replicated across the depression change score outcome and the remission outcome, though not for the response to treatment outcome, and indicate that soldiers who were more severe across multiple areas saw less improvement over time. Ever having been married (married, divorced, separated, or widowed) as compared with never having been married was associated with less improvement in depressive symptoms over time. This finding may be driven in part by the soldiers who were divorced, separated, or widowed rather than the married soldiers, as married individuals generally report less depression than never-married, divorced, separated, and widowed individuals. As discussed, the findings for the initial PHQ-9 score should be interpreted with caution, given that soldiers with higher initial scores had an increased likelihood of symptom improvement, as well as a greater likelihood of response to treatment.

As with the PTSD findings, the treatment factor that was consistently significantly associated with all three depression outcomes was therapeutic alliance between the soldier and provider; better soldier-reported therapeutic alliance scores were associated with better depression outcomes. As noted in the results for PTSD, the therapeutic alliance score comes from the DoD/VA-developed Therapeutic Alliance Questionnaire, addressing three patient self-report areas of alliance. The psychometric properties of the measure have not yet been fully measured, nor have recommended cutoffs or interpretation for the score been established. The variable reflects the last therapeutic alliance score measured during the follow-up period. We also found an association between fewer individual mental health care sessions and better depression outcomes, while a larger supply (more than 30 days) of benzodiazepines and more frequent BH care visits per month, including intensive outpatient visits, for any mental health diagnosis were associated with poorer depression outcomes. It should be noted that these latter findings were not replicated across outcomes. These findings were generally inconsistent, and it is difficult to draw conclusions from them. Nevertheless, as with the findings for PTSD, it appeared that the strength of the working relationship as perceived by the soldier is a consistent factor leading to depressive symptom improvement—more so than frequency of visits or number of treatments.

Pretreatment and Treatment Predictors of Anxiety Symptom Outcomes
Pretreatment and Treatment Predictors of Continuous Anxiety Symptom Change
Table 5.4 shows the multivariate findings examining the factors that were associated with differences between the last follow-up GAD-7 score and the initial score for soldiers in the anxiety sample. Full model results are provided in Table B.6 in Appendix B. The "Estimate" column indicates the size and direction of the relationship between the predictor and the outcome. Specifically, a negative number suggests that the predictor was associated with a decreased GAD-7 score between the initial and last scores. Nine pretreatment and three treatment factors emerged as significant predictors of GAD-7 score changes.

All but one of the significant pretreatment variables were associated with a poorer anxiety outcome. Greater PTSD symptom severity; current pain; a past history of sleep disorder or symptoms; a greater number of days between the first and last GAD-7 scores; and being divorced, separated, or widowed (as compared with never having been married) were all associated with poorer anxiety outcomes; we also found a higher likelihood of poorer outcomes for soldiers who identified as black, non-Hispanic; Hispanic; or other races/ethnicities (compared with white, non-Hispanic soldiers). The one predictor that was associated with reduced anxiety scores over time was a higher initial GAD-7 score.

Three treatment factors were significantly associated with the anxiety change score outcome. A better soldier-reported therapeutic alliance between the soldier and his or her provider was the sole factor that was associated with reductions in anxiety symptoms. Two of the treatment factors were associated with poorer anxiety outcomes: a greater than 30-day supply of benzodiazepines (as compared with no supply) and the number of BH direct care visits per month, including IOP visits, for any MH diagnosis. These latter two findings are not surprising, as soldiers who were more severe received more care, including BH direct care visits and prescribed medications.

Table 5.4
Pretreatment and Treatment Predictors of Difference Between Last and Initial GAD-7 Scores Among Soldiers in the Anxiety Multivariate Analysis Sample (n = 2,592), 2016–2017

Variable	Continuous Anxiety (GAD-7) Outcome	
	Estimate [CI]	P-Value
Time covariates:		
Initial score is after index visit	0.02 [−0.56, 0.59]	0.95
Total days between first-last scores	0.01 [0, 0.01]	0.04
Pretreatment		
Marital status		
Divorced, separated, widowed	1.17 [0.24, 2.11]	0.01
Married	0.64 [−0.01, 1.28]	0.05
Never married [reference group]		
Sex		
Female	0.01 [−0.53, 0.54]	0.98
Age		
18–24	0.36 [−0.85, 1.56]	0.56
25–34	0.45 [−0.56, 1.46]	0.38
35–44	0.65 [−0.3, 1.61]	0.18
45–64 [reference group]		
Race/ethnicity		
Black, non-Hispanic	0.92 [0.39, 1.45]	0.00
Hispanic	0.76 [0.12, 1.4]	0.02
Other	1.06 [0.16, 1.95]	0.02
White, non-Hispanic [reference group]		
Pay grade		
E1–E4	0.39 [−0.55, 1.33]	0.42
E5–E6	0.46 [−0.32, 1.24]	0.25
E7–E9	0.17 [−0.69, 1.03]	0.70
Officer/warrant officer [reference group]		
Total deployments	0.13 [−0.05, 0.31]	0.17

Table 5.4—continued

Variable	Continuous Anxiety (GAD-7) Outcome	
	Estimate [CI]	P-Value
Pain, current	0.95 [0.49, 1.41]	0.00
Initial GAD-7 score	−0.69 [−0.76, −0.61]	0.00
PCL-5 score	0.08 [0.06, 0.09]	0.00
Sleep disorder/symptoms, past history	0.97 [0.52, 1.43]	0.00
Treatment		
Therapeutic Alliance Questionnaire score	−0.11 [−0.14, −0.08]	0.00
Individual therapy visits, direct care, primary/secondary diagnosis, per month	0.06 [−0.19, 0.32]	0.63
BH visits, direct care, with IOP, any MH, per month	0.16 [0.08, 0.25]	0.00
Any MH purchased care	0.6 [−0.02, 1.21]	0.06
Benzodiazepine, days' supply		
0 days [reference group]		
1–30 days	0.21 [−0.56, 0.97]	0.60
>30 days	0.76 [0.08, 1.44]	0.03

NOTE: Current = 30 days prior to 1 week after initial symptom score; past history = 1 year to 30 days prior to initial symptom score.

Pretreatment and Treatment Predictors of Response to Treatment for Soldiers with Anxiety

Response was defined by a point reduction of five or more in GAD-7 scores from the initial to the last follow-up and a final follow-up score of 8 or higher. Full model results are provided in Table B.6 in Appendix B. For pretreatment factors, similar to the continuous outcome findings for GAD-7 change scores, more severe PTSD symptoms and current pain were associated with a lower likelihood of a response to treatment, while a higher initial anxiety score was associated with a greater likelihood of a response to treatment. Female soldiers had a greater likelihood of experiencing an anxiety treatment response, but this finding was not replicated by either of the other two outcomes.

None of the significant findings for the treatment factors observed for the change score outcome was replicated by the response to treatment findings. Only one treatment factor was significantly associated with treatment response: The categorical predictor of receipt of 0 to less than 1.5 BH direct care visits per month, including intensive outpatient visits, for any MH diagnosis (compared with receiving 2.5 or more visits) was associated with a lower likelihood of a response to treatment.

Pretreatment and Treatment Predictors of Remission for Soldiers with Anxiety

Remission was defined by a point reduction of five or more in GAD-7 scores from the initial to the last follow-up and a final score of 7 or less. Full model results are provided in Table B.6 in Appendix B. More severe PTSD symptoms, current pain, and a past history of sleep disorder or symptoms were associated with a lower likelihood of remission at follow-up. All three of these findings were replicated by the findings for the continuous outcome of GAD-7 change scores. The findings for more severe PTSD symptoms and current pain were also a replication of the anxiety response findings. An additional finding not observed by the other outcomes was observed: Compared with soldiers who were between the ages of 45 and 64, those between the ages of 35 and 44 had a lower likelihood of experiencing remission at follow-up.

Two treatment factors were significantly associated with the anxiety remission outcome. A better soldier-reported therapeutic alliance between the soldier and his or her provider was associated with a greater likelihood of remission. In addition, the number of BH direct care visits per month, including IOP visits, for any MH diagnosis was associated with a lower likelihood of remission. Both of these findings for remission replicated findings observed for the continuous outcome for GAD-7 change scores.

Summary of Models to Predict Anxiety Symptom Outcomes

Our findings generally suggested that reports of more severe BH symptoms were associated with worse anxiety outcomes over time. A past history of sleep disorder or symptoms, greater PTSD symptom severity, current pain, and a greater length of time between first and last GAD-7 scores were associated with poorer anxiety outcomes, with the PTSD severity and pain predictor findings replicated across the three outcomes. Sleep findings were replicated across two outcomes. Our findings also revealed that higher initial anxiety scores were associated with better anxiety outcomes; yet, as discussed, these findings should be interpreted with caution, as those with a higher initial anxiety score had more room to improve over the course of treatment. Demographic factors of race/ethnicity, sex, and marital status were associated with anxiety outcomes, though not consistently across all three outcomes. Poorer anxiety outcomes were associated with being divorced, separated, or widowed (as compared with never having been married); being black non-Hispanic, Hispanic, or other race/ethnicity (compared with being white non-Hispanic); and being middle-aged (between age 35 and 44, as compared to being older aged between 45 and 64). Being a woman was associated with better anxiety outcomes at follow-up.

Several treatment factors were associated with anxiety outcomes, though only two findings were replicated across two of the three outcomes. As we found with PTSD and depression outcomes, therapeutic alliance emerged as a significant predictor of better anxiety outcomes, such that a better soldier-reported therapeutic alliance between the soldier and his or her provider was associated with reductions in anxiety symptoms over time and a greater likelihood of remission at follow-up. The finding that poorer anxiety outcomes were associated with a greater number of BH direct care visits per month, including IOP visits, for any MH diagnosis was replicated across two of the anxiety outcomes. As discussed in prior sections, this is likely because those who were more severe would have greater BH service utilization. Findings that more than a 30-day supply of benzodiazepines and fewer BH direct care visits per month, including IOP visits, for any MH diagnosis, were associated with poorer anxiety outcomes over time were not replicated across outcomes.

Summary

When interpreting these findings, it is important to note that, given the observational nature of these data, it is difficult to discern the direction of the observed relationships for the pretreatment and treatment factors. In general, for soldiers in the PTSD sample, greater reported BH symptom severity was associated with better PTSD outcomes over time. Findings for soldiers in the anxiety sample indicated that, in general, greater reported BH symptoms were associated with worse anxiety outcomes over time. Among soldiers in the depression sample, the findings were mixed such that for some outcomes, more severe BH symptoms and poorer functioning were associated with better depression outcomes over time in some instances but worse depression outcomes over time in other instances. Multiple demographic factors emerged from the analyses as well, though these were typically not consistent across the three BH outcomes, nor were they consistent within the three outcomes specific to each BH diagnosis. For example, marital status was associated with two of the three anxiety outcomes, one of the three depression outcomes, and none of the PTSD outcomes. Race/ethnicity, age, and sex effects were also observed for the anxiety outcomes, but none of these factors was associated with PTSD or depression outcomes.

The treatment factors were of main interest in these final models. A consistent treatment factor that was associated with nearly all of the three outcomes within each of the three BH diagnoses was therapeutic alliance, such that a better soldier-reported therapeutic alliance with providers (as measured by the last score of the patient-reported three-item DoD/VA Therapeutic Alliance Questionnaire) was associated with better PTSD, depression, and anxiety outcomes. Multiple reviews of the therapeutic alliance between patients and providers across various areas, such as primary care, physical rehabilitation, and BH, have revealed that a positive and strong therapeutic relationship is an essential component of many types of treatment (Elvins and Green, 2008; Ferreira et al., 2013; Flückiger et al., 2018; Hall et al., 2010; Horvath et al., 2011; Kelley et al., 2014; Martin, Garske, and Davis, 2000). We similarly found this alliance to be the most consistent predictor of improvement over time for PTSD, depression, and anxiety among soldiers receiving BH care in the study samples. Interestingly, this alliance was among the only significant treatment predictors of better BH outcomes.

Other significant treatment factors tended to be associated with poorer behavioral outcomes. More frequent BH care visits, including those for any MH diagnosis, visits that included or did not include IOPs, and visits that included group or individual care, all tended to be associated with poorer BH outcomes over time. Additional treatment utilization may lead to worse outcomes, but it is likely that soldiers who were not improving were subsequently more likely to receive additional care. Although we adjusted our models for severity at initial score, there may have been unmeasured confounders that led to these findings. However, these findings were not consistent across multiple outcomes within specific diagnoses. A notable finding was that a greater than 30-day supply of benzodiazepine medication was associated with poorer PTSD, depression, and anxiety outcomes, including within multiple outcomes for each diagnosis. Clinical practice guidelines and review papers of effective treatments of PTSD, depression, and anxiety generally suggest that the use of benzodiazepines should be limited, closely monitored, used in treatment-resistant cases only, and considered carefully if a patient has a history of substance use disorders (American Psychiatric Association, 2015; Bandelow, Michaelis, and Wedekind, 2017; Bandelow et al., 2008; VA and DoD, 2017). However, patients in multiple BH and primary care settings are given multiple months' supplies of these drugs (Guina et al., 2015; Kroll et al., 2016; Valenstein et al., 2004).

CHAPTER SIX

Trajectories of PTSD, Depression, and Anxiety Symptom Change

In this chapter, we report on our analyses to identify different trajectories of improvement among soldiers in the PTSD, depression, and anxiety samples based on the LCA. These analyses use the trajectory analysis sample (as described in Chapter Two). Specifically, we used the restriction of requiring at least three symptom scores to ensure that we had at least three data points per soldier to estimate a trajectory. To maximize the number of soldiers included in these trajectory detection models, the analyses started with the total sample of soldiers in each diagnosis, regardless of missing predictor variables. The final samples were, however, restricted to soldiers with at least three symptom scores over time. We also describe the likelihood of the different treatment variables being associated with the observed trajectory class. For each of these bivariate associations, the analyses were restricted to cases in which the specific treatment variables were not missing. Based on our analyses, key findings in this chapter include the following:

- Across diagnoses, trajectories showing symptom improvement included fewer soldiers than trajectories showing no improvement.
- Soldiers with PTSD or depression with no improvement tended to have more care utilization, while increased utilization was associated with improvement in soldiers with anxiety.
- Therapeutic alliance and receipt of benzodiazepines had inconsistent associations with symptom change trajectories across PTSD, depression, and anxiety.

Trajectories of PTSD Symptom Change

Of the 3,264 soldiers in the PTSD sample, 2,820 had at least three symptom scores and were included in these analyses. Five trajectory groups (typically referred to as *classes*; we refer to them as *trajectories* here for simplicity) produced the best model fit (sample sizes: 22, 270, 19, 1,068, and 1,441). The first and third trajectories included less than 1 percent of the sample; in the interest of identifying a small number of broad groups for the purposes of characterizing most of the sample into trajectories, we considered these cases to be outliers and dropped them from the sample for reanalysis. For the analysis of the remaining outlier-free sample of 2,779 soldiers, the best model fit resulted in four trajectories (sample sizes: 330, 1,173, 1,151, and 125; see Figure 6.1).

The four trajectories varied based on initial PTSD symptom severity and improvement over time. We named the first trajectory "severe symptoms and improvement" because it included soldiers who started with severe PTSD symptoms and improved markedly over time. This trajectory shows a large improvement (slope = −0.274), equivalent to a 27-point decrease in PCL-5 score after 100 days. This trajectory included only 5 percent of the sample. We named the second trajectory "severe symptoms and no improvement" because it included soldiers who started with severe PTSD symptoms but who did not improve markedly over time. The observed decrease was equivalent to a 1.4-point decrease in PCL-5 score after 100 days (slope = −0.014). A large portion of the sample (41 percent) was in this trajectory.

We named the third trajectory "moderate symptoms and no improvement" because it included soldiers who started with moderate PTSD symptoms (PCL-5 score

Figure 6.1
Four PTSD Symptom Trajectories Among Soldiers in the PTSD Trajectory Analysis Sample (n = 2,779), 2016–2017

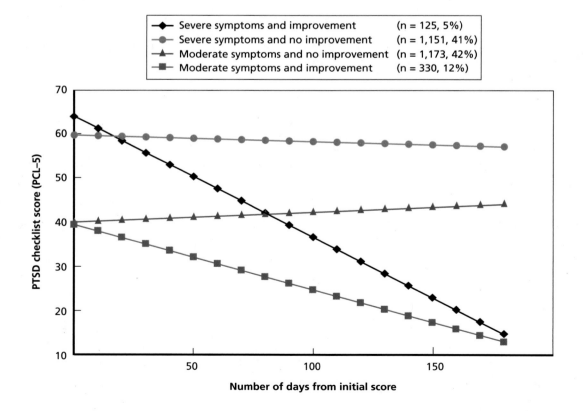

around 40) and did not improve (slope = 0.023, equivalent to a 2.3-point *increase* in PCL-5 score after 100 days). Notably, this trajectory included the highest proportion of soldiers (42 percent). The last trajectory, "moderate symptoms and improvement," also had a moderate starting PCL-5 score (around 40) but showed improvement (slope = 0.145, equivalent to a 15-point decrease in PCL-5 score after 100 days). This trajectory included 12 percent of the sample. Less than one-fifth (17 percent) of soldiers were included in the two trajectories that showed improvement over time.

To investigate the potential predictors of the observed trajectories, we conducted exploratory analyses to assess how each trajectory group varied on treatment variables (see Table 6.1). The pretreatment variables (i.e., demographic and risk variables) were included in the analyses only to identify trajectories; these analyses focused on treatment variables. Nearly all of the treatment variables differed significantly across trajectories. Overall, some patterns emerged:

- Soldiers in the severe symptom trajectories, particularly the trajectory with no improvement, were more likely to have higher utilization (e.g., individual and group psychotherapy visits per month, direct care BH visits, direct outpatient visits).
- Soldiers in the trajectories with no improvement, particularly those starting with more severe symptoms, were most likely to have been dispensed more than 30 days of benzodiazepines.
- Soldiers with severe symptoms and no improvement were most likely to receive both antidepressant treatment and psychotherapy, while soldiers with moderate symptoms and improvement were most likely to receive psychotherapy without antidepressants.
- Soldiers in the trajectories that reflected improvement reported a better therapeutic alliance with their providers (patient-reported DoD/VA Therapeutic Alliance Questionnaire).
- Soldiers in the trajectories with severe symptoms were more likely to have received purchased care as part of their MH care.

Trajectories of Depression Symptom Change

Of the 3,801 soldiers in the depression sample, 3,394 had at least three symptom scores and were included in the analysis. The best-fitting model produced four trajectories (sample sizes: 1,146, 103, 1,525, and 620; see Figure 6.2). For depression, initial PHQ-9 scores were similar for all trajectories, but the four trajectories differed in terms of the amount of symptom improvement. We named the first trajectory "no improvement." Not only was there no improvement, but soldiers in this trajectory showed a potential for symptoms worsening over time (slope = +0.008, or a 0.8-point increase

Table 6.1
Predictors of Membership in PTSD Symptom Trajectories Among Soldiers in the PTSD Trajectory Analysis Sample (n = 2,779), 2016–2017

Treatment Variables	Trajectory Percentage or Mean (SD)				P-Value
	Severe Symptoms and Improvement	Severe Symptoms and No Improvement	Moderate Symptoms and No Improvement	Moderate Symptoms and Improvement	
Any psychotherapy, no antidepressants (%)	17.6	12.3	19.1	24.9	0.000
Any evidence-based therapy (%)	36.8	36.4	35.7	33.9	0.865
Therapeutic Alliance Questionnaire score: mean (SD)	25.7 (6.5)	23.3 (7.0)	24.3 (6.2)	25.3 (6.5)	0.000
Group therapy visits, direct care, primary diagnosis, per month (%)					0.000
≥1 visits	15.2	21.4	11.8	14.8	
0 visits	84.8	78.6	88.2	85.3	
Individual therapy visits, all care, any MH, per month (%)					0.000
0–<3 visits	70.4	64.8	75.4	79.1	
3–4 visits	18.4	20.8	14.7	11.8	
>4 visits	11.2	14.4	10.0	9.1	
Outpatient visits, direct care, primary/secondary diagnosis: mean (SD)	11.4 (12.5)	14.0 (14.8)	12.6 (13.3)	12.3 (12.6)	0.028
BH visits, direct care with IOP, any MH per month: mean (SD)	4.0 (3.1)	4.2 (3.1)	3.4 (2.6)	3.5 (3.2)	0.000
BH visits, direct care without IOP, primary diagnosis per month: mean (SD)	1.8 (1.3)	2.1 (1.6)	1.8 (1.3)	1.6 (1.4)	0.000
BH visits, direct care, without IOP, any MH, per month (%)					0.000
0–<1.5 visits	6.4	13.8	17.8	20.3	
1.5–<2.5 visits	35.2	26.9	33.9	31.5	
≥2.5 visits	58.4	59.3	48.3	48.2	

Table 6.1—continued

Treatment Variables	Trajectory Percentage or Mean (SD)				
	Severe Symptoms and Improvement	Severe Symptoms and No Improvement	Moderate Symptoms and No Improvement	Moderate Symptoms and Improvement	P-Value
Visits in 90 days, primary/ secondary diagnosis, score before intake: mean (SD)	6.6 (7.1)	7.4 (8.1)	6.9 (7.8)	6.6 (5.8)	0.345
Any MH purchased care (%)	23.2	23.3	15.9	11.5	0.000
Benzodiazepines, days' supply (%)					0.000
No days	81.6	76.5	81.3	88.8	
1–30 days	9.6	11.2	8.8	5.8	
31–180 days	8.8	12.3	9.9	5.5	
SSRI/SNRI/antidepressant and psychotherapy (%)	68.8	73.1	66.6	58.2	0.000

NOTES: The mean differences for therapeutic alliance are statistically significant. However, we do not have data to interpret the extent to which these differences are clinically significant.

in PHQ-9 score after 100 days). Notably, this was the second-largest class, accounting for 34 percent of the sample. The second trajectory showed the most marked improvement in depression symptoms (referred to as a "large improvement"; slope = −0.18, or an 18-point decrease in PHQ-9 score after 100 days) but represented only 3 percent of the sample.

The third trajectory, named "small improvement," was the largest of the four, accounting for 45 percent of the sample. Soldiers in this trajectory showed only a small decrease in depression symptoms (slope = −0.02, or a two-point decrease in PHQ-9 score after 100 days). We named the fourth trajectory "moderate improvement," as soldiers in this trajectory showed a moderate decrease in scores (slope = −0.08, or an eight-point decrease in PHQ-9 score after 100 days). This trajectory included 18 percent of the sample.

We conducted exploratory analyses to assess how each trajectory group varied on treatment variables (see Table 6.2). Nearly all the treatment variables differed significantly across trajectories. Overall, some patterns emerged:

- Soldiers with no improvement had higher utilization for some aspects of treatment (e.g., individual and group psychotherapy, MH outpatient visits).

Figure 6.2
Four Depression Symptom Trajectories Among Soldiers in the Depression Trajectory Analysis Sample (n = 3,394), 2016–2017

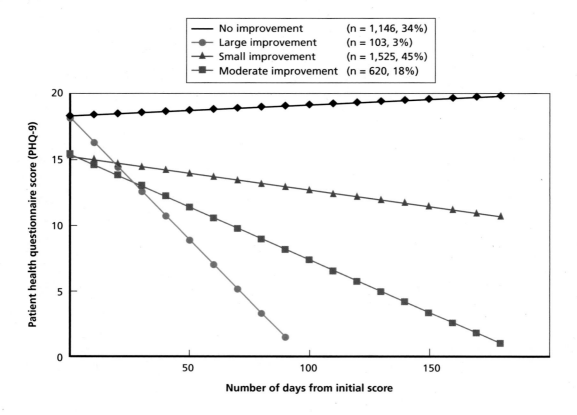

- Soldiers with no improvement were most likely to have more than a 30-day supply of benzodiazepines.
- Soldiers with no improvement were most likely to receive both antidepressant treatment and psychotherapy and least likely to receive psychotherapy alone with no antidepressant.
- Soldiers in the trajectories who had small and moderate improvement reported higher therapeutic alliance (patient-reported DoD/VA Therapeutic Alliance Questionnaire) with their providers than soldiers in the trajectories with no and large improvement.
- Soldiers in the trajectory with no improvement were more likely to have received purchased care as part of their mental health care.

Table 6.2
Predictors of Membership in Depression Symptom Trajectories Among Soldiers in the Trajectory Analysis Depression Sample (n = 3,394), 2016–2017

Treatment Variables	Trajectory Percentage or Mean (SD)				
	No Improvement	Small Improvement	Moderate Improvement	Large Improvement	P-Value
E&M visits, all care, primary diagnosis: mean (SD)	1.6 (2.3)	1.5 (2.4)	1.7 (2.4)	1.8 (2.2)	0.367
Psychotherapy visits, no antidepressants (%)	10.4	12.2	15.8	24.3	0.000
Therapeutic Alliance Questionnaire score: mean (SD)	22.4 (7.4)	24.0 (6.1)	25.6 (5.9)	23.6 (7.2)	0.000
Group therapy visits, direct care, primary diagnosis, per month: mean (SD)	0.2 (1.0)	0.1 (0.4)	0.1 (0.3)	0.1 (0.6)	0.001
Individual therapy visits, direct care, type 1 provider, any MH, per month (%)					0.000
0–<2 visits	41.0	50.2	53.9	46.6	
2–<4 visits	42.7	40.1	37.3	40.8	
≥4 visits	16.3	9.7	8.9	12.6	
Outpatient visits, all care, any MH: mean (SD)	25.6 (21.7)	19.8 (18.1)	17.2 (14.2)	13.3 (11.0)	0.000
BH visits, direct care, with IOP, primary/secondary diagnosis per month: mean (SD)	2.0 (2.3)	1.8 (1.8)	1.9 (1.9)	2.0 (2.1)	0.128
BH visits, direct care, without IOP, primary diagnosis per month: mean (SD)	1.2 (1.4)	1.3 (1.3)	1.5 (1.5)	1.4 (1.2)	0.000
BH visits, direct care, with IOP, primary diagnosis, per month (%)					0.003
0–<1.5 visits	66.3	64.5	57.7	54.4	
1.5–<2.5 visits	15.5	17.1	20.5	26.2	
≥2.5 visits	18.2	18.4	21.8	19.4	
BH visits, direct care, without IOP, primary diagnosis, per month (%)					0.001
0–<1.5 visits	69.3	66.9	59.8	59.2	

Table 6.2—continued

Treatment Variables	Trajectory Percentage or Mean (SD)				P-Value
	No Improvement	Small Improvement	Moderate Improvement	Large Improvement	
1.5–<2.5 visits	16.6	17.8	21.3	27.2	
≥2.5 visits	14.1	15.3	18.9	13.6	
3+ visits, any MH diagnosis (%)	83.5	86.2	86.6	88.4	0.141
3+ visits, primary diagnosis, type 1 provider (%)	38.1	35.9	41.8	36.9	0.084
Any MH purchased care (%)	25.9	16.2	17.7	19.4	0.000
Benzodiazepine, days' supply (%)					0.000
No days	76.5	856	88.9	90.3	
1–30 days	10.5	6.0	5.7	7.8	
31–180 days	13	8.4	5.5	1.9	
SSRI/SNRI/antidepressant and psychotherapy (%)	89.2	87.1	84.0	71.8	0.000

Trajectories of Anxiety Symptom Change

Of the 4,282 soldiers in the anxiety sample, 3,601 had at least three symptom scores and were included in the analysis. Three trajectories produced the best model fit (sample sizes: 1,615, 1,315, and 671; see Figure 6.3). We named the first trajectory "no improvement," as soldiers in this trajectory had slightly higher starting GAD-7 scores and did not show a decrease in symptoms. In fact, soldiers in this trajectory potentially had a slight increase in the score (slope = +0.005, or a 0.5-point increase in GAD-7 score after 100 days). Notably, this trajectory included the largest proportion of the sample (45 percent). The second trajectory, referred to as "moderate improvement," reflected a moderate decrease in scores (slope = −0.03, or a three-point decrease in GAD-7 score after 100 days) relative to the other trajectories. This trajectory included about one-third of the sample (36 percent). We named the third trajectory "large improvement" because soldiers in this trajectory had the largest decrease in anxiety symptoms (slope = −0.08, or an eight-point decrease in GAD-7 score after 100 days). This trajectory included the smallest proportion of the sample (19 percent). Across these trajectories, the initial scores were similar but slightly lower for the two trajectories with improvement over time when compared with the trajectory no improvement.

Figure 6.3
Three Anxiety Symptom Trajectories Among Soldiers in the Anxiety Trajectory Analysis Sample (n = 3,601), 2016–2017

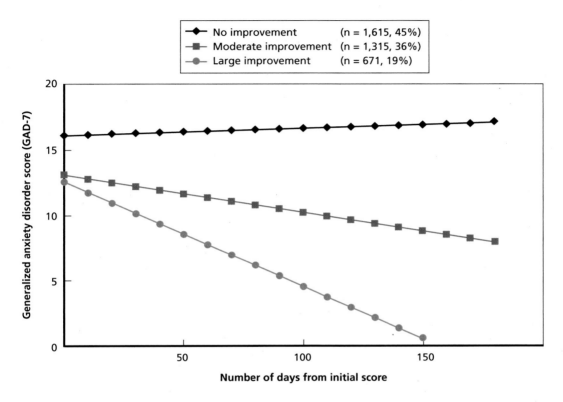

We conducted exploratory analyses to assess how each trajectory group varied in terms of treatment variables (see Table 6.3). Many of the treatment variables differed significantly across trajectories. Unlike the trajectory findings for PTSD and depression, our trajectory analyses for anxiety showed that those in the large-improvement trajectory (19 percent) were most likely to have more than a 30-day supply of benzodiazepines. This group was a small portion of the anxiety sample, and the trajectory analyses do not take into account other pretreatment and treatment variables. Overall, some patterns emerged:

- Soldiers with no improvement had higher utilization for some aspects of treatment (e.g., individual and group psychotherapy, MH outpatient visits).
- Soldiers in the large-improvement trajectory were most likely to have more than a 30-day supply of benzodiazepines, a finding that is inconsistent with our other findings.

Table 6.3
Predictors of Membership in Anxiety Symptom Trajectories Among Soldiers in the Anxiety Trajectory Analysis Sample (n = 3,601), 2016–2017

Treatment Variables	Trajectory Percentage or Mean (SD)			
	No Improvement	Moderate Improvement	Large Improvement	P-Value
E&M visits, all care, primary diagnosis: mean (SD)	1.1 (1.7)	1.0 (1.7)	0.9 (1.5)	0.198
Any psychotherapy, no antidepressants (%)	23.6	19.5	13.8	0.000
Any evidence-based therapy (%)	68.4	72.2	70.3	0.191
Therapeutic Alliance Questionnaire score: mean (SD)	25.8 (5.8)	24.3 (6.1)	23.0 (7.2)	0.000
Group therapy visits, direct care, primary diagnosis, per month: mean (SD)	0.0 (0.3)	0.0 (0.3)	0.1 (0.6)	0.200
Individual therapy visits, direct care, primary diagnosis, per month: mean (SD)	0.8 (0.9)	0.7 (0.8)	0.7 (0.8)	0.017
Individual therapy visits, direct care, primary/ secondary diagnosis, per month: mean (SD)	0.9 (0.9)	0.9 (0.8)	0.9 (0.9)	0.393
BH visits, direct care, with IOP, any MH per month: mean (SD)	2.8 (2.1)	2.8 (2.1)	3.5 (3.0)	0.000
BH visits, direct care, with IOP, any MH, per month (%)				0.000
0–<1.5 visits	23.1	228	18.1	
1.5–<2.5 visits	35.2	35.4	27.6	
≥2.5 visits	41.7	41.8	54.3	
BH visits, direct care, with IOP, primary/ secondary diagnosis, per month (%)				0.026
0–<1.5 visits	60.7	65.7	66.7	
1.5–<2.5 visits	24.6	21.1	19.0	
≥2.5 visits	14.8	13.2	14.8	
Visits in 90 days, primary diagnosis: mean (SD)	2.6 (3.6)	2.6 (3.7)	2.5 (3.4)	0.557
3+ visits, any MH diagnosis, type 2 provider (%)	19.8	19.3	16.8	0.120
3+ visits, primary diagnosis, type 1 provider (%)	33.1	29.7	28.7	0.114
Any MH purchased care (%)	10	11.5	18.8	0.000
Benzodiazepine, days' supply (%)				0.000

Table 6.3—continued

Treatment Variables	Trajectory Percentage or Mean (SD)			
	No Improvement	Moderate Improvement	Large Improvement	P-Value
No days	86.7	81.4	73.6	
1–30 days	5.7	9.0	11.5	
31–180 days	7.6	9.7	14.9	
SSRI/SNRI/antidepressant and psychotherapy (%)	64.1	65.8	72.4	0.000

- Soldiers in the large-improvement trajectory were most likely to receive both antidepressant treatment and psychotherapy and least likely to receive psychotherapy alone.
- Soldiers in the no-improvement trajectory reported a better therapeutic alliance with their providers (patient-reported DoD/VA Therapeutic Alliance Questionnaire).
- Soldiers in the large-improvement trajectory were more likely to have received purchased care as part of their MH care.

Summary

Our analyses of symptom trajectories identified groups of soldiers with varying amounts of improvement in their symptoms over time and often identified trajectories with differing initial symptom severities. Across diagnoses, trajectories that showed symptom improvement included fewer soldiers than trajectories that showed no improvement. For PTSD and depression, soldiers with no improvement tended to have more care utilization. Given the observational nature of these data, it is difficult to discern the direction of this relationship. Although our analyses adjusted for the severity of the initial symptom score, they may not fully account for initial severity or risk of a poorer outcome. Providers may ensure that soldiers with more severe symptoms at the time of the initial score receive more treatment. Furthermore, providers may recommend additional treatment, or treatment adjustment, for soldiers who do not respond to an initial treatment. The treatment variables included in the exploratory models described in this chapter were selected based on treatment predictors that were in our final multivariable models in Chapter Five; therefore, some variables (e.g., type of provider) were not evaluated in these models. On the other hand, for the anxiety sample, more utilization was associated with a decrease in GAD-7 scores. While therapeutic alliance and receipt of benzodiazepines showed relatively consistent relationships with outcomes in our multivariate analyses (Chapter Five), these predictors had inconsistent associations with symptom change trajectories across PTSD, depression, and anxiety.

CHAPTER SEVEN

Summary and Recommendations

In this chapter, we highlight the strengths and limitations of our analyses, highlight our main findings, and provide recommendations for how the Army can continue to improve outcomes for soldiers who receive BH care.

We identified three samples of active-component Army soldiers who received care for PTSD (n = 3,264), depression (n = 3,801), or anxiety (n = 4,282) from the MHS who met the following criteria:

- were seen in specialty BH care in 2016–2017 for the target condition, allowing for a minimum six-month time frame from sample entry
- began a new treatment episode, defined as no specialty BH care associated with the diagnosis in the prior six months
- had a minimal level of symptom severity as measured by the PCL-5, PHQ-9, or GAD-7 (for PTSD, depression, and anxiety, respectively)
- had a second symptom score one to six months later.

We used the identified samples to do the following:

- We characterized the frequency and distribution of follow-up symptom scores as measured for the samples during the six months after the index BH visit.
- We proposed a set of pretreatment and treatment variables as possible predictors of outcome based on the relevant literature. We then carried out a multistep process to select "best-in-class" variables and those that were the best predictors of outcomes to include in the multivariate analyses.
- We described the characteristics of the smaller population of soldiers with data for the selected pretreatment variables, including the frequency of their outpatient visits, and their comorbidities.
- We examined how the soldiers in our multivariate analysis samples compared with soldiers who had BH care for one of the three target diagnoses but did not meet the other criteria for sample inclusion.

- We explored the symptom score data for soldiers with at least three symptom scores to document trajectory patterns of change in score over the subsequent six months.

Strengths and Limitation of the Analyses

The analyses presented in this report have several strengths. We developed a linked data set, drawing together ten data sources, which allowed us to characterize many aspects of soldiers and their care. Our multivariate analyses examined a lengthy list of potential predictors, including pretreatment and treatment variables, with detailed variable selection steps to ensure parsimonious models. We screened out variables with little variability and tested collinear variables, retaining only the most influential ones. The variable selection process also involved evaluating in groups variables within similar constructs, a process that aimed to avoid spurious correlation that could have led to the removal of some important predictors. The trajectory analysis also provided a supplemental way to assess improvement in soldiers' outcomes. Finally, we conducted our analyses across three target diagnoses and three symptom score outcomes, allowing us to identify consistent patterns across analyses.

At the same time, the work presented in this report also has several limitations. The sample studied was limited to soldiers receiving BH care with a new treatment episode, a minimal level of symptom severity, and at least one follow-up symptom score in one to six months. Our results do not include those who received Army BH care but did not have any symptom scores or less than two scores or had a lower level of symptom severity at first visit. Therefore, our results may not generalize to these other populations. Although we examined a lengthy list of variables, there were some variables that we could not evaluate because they were not included in the data (e.g., personality traits, perceived quality of life, lifetime history of trauma).

Furthermore, some variables may not adequately capture the treatment delivered. For example, we examined a provider-entered variable for type of evidence-based psychotherapy, but it was not predictive of outcomes—a surprising result, given the research support for these therapies in reducing symptoms. However, a limitation of the variable used in this study is that it comes from the BHDP and is an optional provider-reported checklist of therapies provided to the patient. These data may overrepresent or underrepresent the provision of evidence-based therapy and do not indicate the frequency of sessions. A prior assessment of the use of evidence-based psychotherapy in direct care for PTSD and depression (and based on medical record abstraction) across service branches found that rates of receipt of evidence-based psychotherapy could improve (45 percent and 30 percent, respectively, among service members who receive any psychotherapy) (Hepner, Roth, et al., 2017). The lack of association could be related to the quality of the variable (e.g., providers indicated delivering a psychotherapy but did not deliver it with adequate fidelity or the soldier did not receive an adequate number of psychotherapy sessions) or the level of missing data in some variables.

Another variable that was important in this study was the total days' supply of benzodiazepines dispensed over the soldier's follow-up period. The variable does not capture the pattern of how the medication was dispensed over time. Thus, the variable likely captures soldiers who have longer-term use of benzodiazepines versus shorter, more limited prescriptions. There may be some unique circumstances when a soldier may receive a larger supply of medications (e.g., at separation from service when transition to VA care may take some time). An evaluation of the greater-than-30-days' supply would need to consider several variables, such as dosage, time over which the medication was dispensed, and other pertinent diagnoses. The analysis of these factors was beyond the scope of this study and was a limitation.

Some limitations regarding therapeutic alliance should be noted. This variable is a patient-reported measure, and the clinician may have a different perspective of the alliance. The therapeutic alliance measure used by the Army is early in its development, and there are no published analyses of its psychometric properties. In addition, our analyses used the last available therapeutic alliance score. In our study samples, approximately 50 percent had their last therapeutic alliance score on the same date as the last symptom score. Some soldiers had earlier therapeutic alliance scores, but not all. If we were to have required that the therapeutic alliance score be prior to the last symptom score, it would have further limited our effective sample size. In addition, we selected the last score in part because this was the score the Army had used in its preliminary analyses of outcomes. Use of the last therapeutic alliance score could have biased our results because patients who are feeling better may be more likely to report a strong alliance with their provider, thus increasing the likelihood of finding an association with the last symptom score.

The observational nature of the data limited our ability to draw causal links between the predictors and outcomes. In addition, even with careful variable selection, there is always the possibility of remaining collinearity, which could produce biased estimates of the association between an outcome and some predictors. With the time span between the initial and last score varying across soldiers, there is also the possibility of such a time variable moderating (or interacting with) the association between predictors and outcomes. Similarly, the use of the outcome as the change from initial score to the last score does not capture all of the changes that occurred in the interim. The symptom scores used to select the sample were based on one initial elevated score, and such scores can vary even for an individual soldier, leading to the possibility that the high initial score used to select the sample was an outlier. This can make the subsequent scores observed over time regress toward the mean (or the true outcome score), and the change score could be an artifact of an outlying initial score. For the trajectory analysis, there is always the possibility of a nonlinear trajectory for individual soldiers, thus limiting the assumptions in our analysis, but with the data structure and the possibly large number of times when scores were observed, inference and interpretation of a nonlinear trajectory model can be complex. Also, because some of the characteristics used as predictors of the trajectories vary over time, some of the observed relationships could be explained by reverse causation.

Despite these limitations, this report provides thorough analyses of patterns of symptom score data and identifies potentially important aspects of treatment that were associated with improved outcomes. The remainder of this chapter highlights the main findings from our study, followed by recommendations to improve Army BH care.

Findings

BHDP Is Widely Used to Track PTSD, Depression, and Anxiety Symptoms, but There Are Opportunities to Expand Symptom Tracking

We found consistent patterns of outcome monitoring related to BHDP implementation and uptake across the three soldier samples. It was generally the case that soldiers in all three samples received more scores the longer they were in treatment and the longer the period between their first and last symptom measure scores. This suggests that BHDP has been widely implemented and that soldiers were routinely receiving scores during BH visits. However, there were some areas for improvement. First, some soldiers in each of the three samples had BH visits after their last symptom measure score, suggesting that BH visits occurred without the provider using symptom measures. Thus, a soldier's last score was not necessarily a measure of his or her symptoms at treatment end. In addition, soldiers in the anxiety sample were less likely than soldiers in the PTSD and depression samples to receive multiple scores; this pattern was more apparent when we considered soldiers with 16 or more BH visits and noted that double the number of anxiety sample soldiers received very few scores (i.e., two or three) compared with soldiers in the PTSD and depression samples. Army monitoring of anxiety symptoms was implemented after monitoring for PTSD and depression, so these results could reflect differing stages of implementation. Lastly, using BHDP data, we applied the NQF-endorsed measures of depression response and remission that are currently used in civilian populations to monitor depression outcomes. However, there are significant differences in the technical specifications used by the Army versus NQF (e.g., the Army limits the measures to soldiers with an NTE, requires a second score, and uses different response and remission definitions). These differences between the Army methodology for computing depression response and remission measures and the NQF-endorsed measures make comparison between Army and civilian care difficult.

Stronger Patient-Reported Therapeutic Alliance Was Associated with Improved PTSD, Depression, and Anxiety Outcomes

Despite using methods to identify "best-in-class" pretreatment and treatment factors that were associated with clinical outcomes, we found that no pretreatment variables were consistently associated with outcomes. That is, no demographic or risk factors were consistently associated with all three targeted outcomes within a diagnosis (i.e., change scores, response to treatment, and remission) or across diagnoses. However, one treatment factor was consistently associated with outcomes both within and between diagnoses: therapeutic alliance. A stronger soldier-reported therapeutic alliance was associated with decreased PTSD, depression, and anxiety symptoms; PTSD and depression response to treatment; and PTSD, depression, and anxiety remission. This factor emerged even when controlling for such factors as the number of sessions and the number of different treatments received, indicating that a perceived strong working relationship between soldiers and their providers may be an essential component of symptom improvement regardless of BH target.

Increased Supply of Benzodiazepines Was Associated with Worse PTSD, Depression, and Anxiety Outcomes

Besides therapeutic alliance, no other treatment factor was consistently associated with improved outcomes over time within or between diagnoses. However, it was generally the case that a greater days' supply of benzodiazepine medication (i.e., more than a 30-days' supply as compared to no supply) was associated with poorer PTSD, depression, and anxiety outcomes. More specifically, this factor was associated with a poorer change score outcome and less likelihood of a response to treatment for the PTSD sample, a poorer change score outcome for the depression sample, and a poorer change score outcome for the anxiety sample. High rates of comorbid PTSD in the depression and anxiety samples (approximately 40 percent) may have contributed to observing this relationship across all samples. We cannot assume that a prescription or filling of a larger supply of a medication indicates a greater level of use. Our study was unable to assess whether the soldiers used benzodiazepines as prescribed, but the soldiers who had a greater days' supply of the drug were the ones who experienced poorer outcomes. The findings were consistent enough across diagnoses to conclude that having a larger supply of these medications indicated poorer outcomes over time. Our trajectory analyses for anxiety, however, showed that those in the large improvement trajectory (19 percent) were most likely to receive more than a 30-day supply of benzodiazepines. This group was a small portion of the anxiety sample, and the trajectory analyses do not take into account other pretreatment and treatment variables. Further research is needed to determine whether soldiers whose symptoms are less likely to improve in treatment are given these medications or whether being given these medications leads to impediments in symptom improvement.

Many Soldiers' Trajectories of Change Did Not Demonstrate Improvement

Outcome quality measures currently tracked by the Army—response to treatment and remission—show improvement in one to six months after the initial elevated score for those soldiers with at least one additional follow-up score but also highlight a need to continue to improve the effectiveness of Army BH care. According to symptom score data for the samples in our study, the rates of response or remission based on the Army methodology were 35 percent for PTSD, 45 percent for depression, and 41 percent for anxiety. Of note is an NQF-endorsed measure of depression response and remission used in commercial, Medicare, and Medicaid populations that uses technical specifications that differ from the Army's (NQF, 2018). These differences prevent comparison of the Army outcome rates of performance with the civilian rates. We also conducted analyses to identify groups of soldiers based on their pattern of symptom change over time (i.e., trajectories). These analyses identified three or four different trajectories for each sample. Across these samples, the majority of soldiers with PTSD (83 percent) were included in a trajectory that did not demonstrate improvement in their symptoms. Among patients with depression, 79 percent were included in a trajectory that showed no (34 percent) or small improvement (45 percent), and 45 percent of the anxiety sample were in a trajectory that showed no improvement. Exploring predictors of the trajectories yielded mixed results. Often, predictors that captured increased utilization were associated with a lack of improvement, but because of the observational nature of the data, it was difficult to ascertain the direction of causality. Additional treatment utilization may lead to worse outcomes, but it is likely that soldiers who were not improving were subsequently more likely to receive additional care. Although we adjusted our models for severity at initial score, there may have been unmeasured confounders that led to these findings.

Recommendations and Policy Implications

Recommendation 1: Provide Feedback on Therapeutic Alliance and Guidance to Providers on How to Strengthen Alliance with Their Patients

Stronger therapeutic alliance is associated with improved outcomes, a robust finding that has been observed in prior literature. Giving providers, clinic leads, or MTFs information about how soldiers perceive their alliances with providers may provide an important early indicator on how treatment is going. At an individual patient level, providers can address difficulties in the therapeutic relationship directly with the patient and use this information to repair the relationship or address concerns about treatment that the patient may have. Provider training on how to assess therapeutic alliance and respond appropriately when a patient rates the alliance as weak may be a key strategy in minimizing treatment dropout and improving outcomes. Our analyses were somewhat limited by relying on the last therapeutic alliance score, which was frequently assessed at the same time as the last symptom score, potentially biasing results by increasing the association between these two variables. Therefore, we recommend that Army ensure that therapeutic alliance is routinely assessed early in treatment. This will ensure that the results of the measure are actionable during treatment for the clinician and that these analyses can be replicated using alliance scores that are collected prior to the last symptom outcome score.

Recommendation 2: Expand Tracking and Feedback on Benzodiazepine Prescribing

One of the most consistent findings in our analyses was that soldiers who were dispensed more days of benzodiazepines—more than 30 days—were more likely to have worse outcomes. The clinical practice guideline for PTSD cautions against using benzodiazepines as monotherapy or augmentation therapy for the treatment of PTSD (VA and DoD, 2017), and these medications have been identified as potentially harmful in this population. In 2018, the Defense Health Agency initiated the PTS Provider Prescribing Profile to track benzodiazepine prescribing among providers who treat PTSD and acute stress disorder (Military Health System Communications Office, 2018). Results are monitored and shared with MTF commanders. The Army's Behavioral Health Service Line is also tracking benzodiazepines and atypical antipsychotic prescriptions for PTSD (Woolaway-Bickel, 2019). Data on benzodiazepine prescribing could also be provided to clinic leadership and individual providers as a potential approach to improve patient outcomes, including response to treatment and remission metrics. Additional work could be conducted to identify the duration of benzodiazepine use that may lead to worse outcomes, but our analyses suggest that more than a 30-day supply is associated with worse outcomes.

Recommendation 3: Increase Provider Use of Measurement-Based Behavioral Health Care

The Army continues to expand and monitor the use of BHDP in BH care. Our analyses were restricted to soldiers who had at least two symptom scores (among other eligibility criteria), so our analyses do not include soldiers who received BH care with a target diagnoses but were not assessed more than once. A 2016 survey of BH providers suggested that 76 percent of Army BH providers screened for PTSD or depression using a validated measure, but only 59 percent reported using symptom data to inform treatment (Hepner, Farris, et al., 2017). Indeed, across our samples of soldiers with at least two scores, only 73 percent of those with PTSD, 77 percent of those with depression, and 68 percent of those with anxiety had more than three scores over their follow-up period, which could have been up to six months. Measurement-based care involves repeatedly collecting outcome data and using those data to inform treatment decisions throughout the course of treatment (Fortney et al., 2016). These data provide timely feedback to providers about patient progress, allowing providers to quickly identify patients who are not improving or deteriorating (Boswell et al., 2015). It remains possible that many Army providers are measuring scores at a frequency that does not allow for this "real-time" adjustment in treatment. Providers may view measurement-based care as valuable but may still face implementation challenges (Jensen-Doss et al., 2018). As the Army continues to expand the use of BHDP and collection of symptom measures, supporting providers in frequent collection and use of this information may also be an important strategy for improving BH outcomes.

Directions for Future Research

The analyses presented in this report provide results that can guide the Army in improving outcomes for soldiers who receive BH care. These analyses also raised several questions that could be addressed in future research:

- *Identify quality of care measures that can help providers focus on aspects of treatment that have the highest likelihood of improving soldier outcomes (sometimes referred to as "driver metrics.")* These analyses would target therapeutic alliance and supply of benzodiazepines to identify detailed specifications for tracking metrics to assess these variables that are associated with treatment outcomes.
- *Evaluate whether refinements in the definitions of response to treatment and remission currently used by the Army could improve assessment of significant symptom improvement and increases in psychosocial functioning.* Our analyses highlighted that several soldiers who receive at least some Army BH care are excluded from the outcome measures. For example, current Army specifications exclude soldiers who are not in a new episode of treatment, those with symptom scores that do not meet the severity threshold, and those without a follow-up score. Expanding inclusion, or developing alternative metrics, may provide more opportunities to more thoroughly monitor the effectiveness of Army BH care. Further, modifications to measure specifications could also improve the ability to compare Army performance with civilian care settings.
- *Explore the utility of alternative approaches to monitoring Army outcome measures (i.e., response to treatment and remission).* This could include tracking these metrics stratified by populations of interest (e.g., broken out by demographic characteristics or those on a medical evaluation board). Stratified reporting of outcome measures has been suggested as an alternative to complex case-mix adjustment models.
- *Explore the utility of expanding Army BH outcome monitoring beyond symptom measures.* The Army is a leader in monitoring outcomes of BH care. Thus far, this monitoring has focused on symptom measures. This is a logical focus, as symptoms are the most proximal outcome of BH care, and most likely to be improved by high-quality care. However, the Army could explore monitoring other out-

comes of BH care. Potential targets could include indicators of readiness, functioning, or quality of life.

- *Develop and evaluate more effective treatments for PTSD, depression, and anxiety disorders.* Our analyses add to existing recent literature that has called for more effective treatments, particularly for service members with PTSD. The observed rates of response to treatment and remission highlight the continued need for more effective treatments within both Army and non-Army settings.

Variables Used in the Multivariate Models

Table A.1
Pretreatment and Treatment Variables Included in the Analyses

Variable	Variable Description
Pretreatment Demographic Data and Characteristics	
Demographic data at initial score:	
Marital status	Marital status [Married; divorced, separated, or widowed; never married]
Sex	Sex [Male; female]
Age	Age [18–24; 25–34; 35–44; 45–64]
Race/ethnicity	Race/ethnicity [White, non-Hispanic; black, non-Hispanic; Hispanic; other]
Service-related characteristics at initial score:	
Years of service	Total years of active military service
Pay grade	Pay grade [E1–E4; E5–E6; E7–E9; officer/warrant officer]
Total deployments	Total number of deployments
Months deployed	Total months deployed
Warrior Transition Unit (WTU)	Warrior Transition Unit (self-report)
Medical Evaluation Board (MEB)	Disability evaluation in progress (self-report)
Separation in progress	Administrative separation in progress (self-report)
Symptoms (30 days prior to 1 week after initial score):	
General distress (BASIS score)	Behavior and Symptom Identification Scale score
Suicide risk (C-SSRS, current score)	Columbia Suicide Severity Rating Scale, current score

Table A.1—continued

Variable	Variable Description
Alcohol consumption (AUDIT-C score)	Alcohol Use Disorders Identification Test–Concise
Insomnia severity (ISI score)	Insomnia Severity Index score
Time to fall asleep	On average, how long did it take you to fall asleep in the past month? [0–15 min; 16–30 min; 31–45 min; 46–60 min; more than 60 min]
Hours of sleep	On average, how many hours did you sleep each night during the past month? [Less than 4 hrs; 4–5 hrs; 6–7 hrs; 8–9 hrs; 10 or more hrs]
Daytime sleepiness	Do you frequently feel that you need to take a nap during the day? [Yes/No]
Function	Overall, how difficult is it for you to do your work, take care of things at home, or get along with other people? [Not at all; somewhat difficult; very difficult; extremely difficult]
Function, personal/social (WRAIR PSF score)	Walter Reed Functional Impairment Scale, personal/social functioning score
Function, occupational (WRAIR OF score)	Walter Reed Functional Impairment Scale, occupational functioning score
CSI score	Couple Satisfaction Index score
Pain, current	Are you experiencing pain now? [Yes/No]
Initial PCL-5 score	Initial elevated PTSD Checklist for DSM-5 score ($\geq$29) within 30 days of the index visit and in the PSTD sample
Initial PHQ-9 score	Initial elevated Patient Health Questionnaire, 9-item scale score ($\geq$10) within 30 days of the index visit and in the depression sample
Initial GAD-7 score	Initial elevated Generalized Anxiety Disorder, 7-item scale score ($\geq$10) within 30 days of the index visit and in the anxiety sample
PHQ-9 score	Patient Health Questionnaire, 9-item scale score for PTSD or anxiety sample
GAD-7 score	Generalized Anxiety Disorder, 7-item scale score for PTSD or depression sample
PCL-5 score	PTSD Checklist for DSM-5 score for depression or anxiety sample

Past history of diagnosis (>1 month to 1 year prior to initial score):

Depression, past history	Diagnosis of depression
PTSD, past history	Diagnosis of posttraumatic stress disorder
Anxiety, past history	Diagnosis of anxiety
Sleep disorder/symptoms, past history	Diagnosis of sleep disorder/symptoms

Table A.1—continued

Variable	Variable Description
Personality disorder, past history	Diagnosis of personality disorder
Substance use disorder, past history	Diagnosis of substance use disorder (alcohol or drug)
Drug use disorder, past history	Diagnosis of drug use disorder
Alcohol use disorder, past history	Diagnosis of alcohol use disorder
Traumatic brain injury (TBI), past history	Diagnosis of TBI
Dysthymia, past history	Diagnosis of dysthymia
Current diagnosis (1 month prior to 1 week after initial score):	
Depression, current	Diagnosis of depression (and in PTSD or anxiety sample)
PTSD, current	Diagnosis of posttraumatic stress disorder (and in depression or anxiety sample)
Anxiety, current	Diagnosis of anxiety (and in PTSD or depression sample)
Sleep disorder/symptoms, current	Diagnosis of sleep disorder/symptoms
Personality disorder, current	Diagnosis of personality disorder
Substance use disorder, current	Diagnosis of substance use disorder (alcohol or drug)
Drug use disorder, current	Diagnosis of drug use disorder
Alcohol use disorder, current	Diagnosis of alcohol use disorder
TBI, current	Diagnosis of TBI
Dysthymia, current	Diagnosis of dysthymia
Past history or current diagnosis (1 year prior to 1 week after initial score):	
MH comorbidity index	Mental health comorbidity index, number of diagnosis categories (up to 7): acute stress disorder/PTSD; adjustment disorder; anxiety disorder; depression; alcohol use/dependence; drug use/dependence; TBI
Current psychotropic medication (in 1 month prior to initial score):	
Psychotropic medication, current	Flag for taking a psychotropic medication: antidepressant; hypnotic/sedative/anxiolytic; antipsychotic; mood stabilizer/anticonvulsant; stimulant; prazosin; other
Past health care utilization (>1 month to 1 year prior to initial score):	
Non-MH outpatient visits	Number of non–mental health outpatient visits, direct and purchased care

Table A.1—continued

Variable	Variable Description
MH outpatient visits	Number of mental health outpatient visits, direct and purchased care
Outpatient visits	Number of outpatient encounters, direct and purchased care
Any MH inpatient discharge	Flag for any mental health inpatient discharge, direct or purchased care
Past health care utilization (4 months prior to initial score):	
Non-MH outpatient visits, prior 4 months	Number of non–mental health outpatient visits, direct and purchased care
MH outpatient visits, prior 4 months	Number of mental health outpatient visits, direct and purchased care
Treatment Variables	
Time covariates:	
Initial score after intake	Flag for initial elevated score occurred after intake visit
Days between first-last scores, categorical	Categorical number of days between initial elevated and last scores [30–60 days; 61–90 days; 91–120 days; 121–150 days; 151–180 days]
Total days between first-last scores	Number days between initial elevated and last scores
Treatment between initial and last scores (unless otherwise specified):	
E&M visits:	
E&M visits, all care, any MH	Number of evaluation and management visits, direct care and purchased care: any mental health diagnosis
E&M visits, direct care, any MH	Number of evaluation and management visits, direct care: any mental health diagnosis
E&M visits, all care, primary diagnosis	Number of evaluation and management visits, direct care and purchased care: target condition primary diagnosis
E&M visits, direct care, primary diagnosis	Number of evaluation and management visits, direct care: target condition primary diagnosis
E&M visits, all care, primary/ secondary diagnosis	Number of evaluation and management visits, direct care and purchased care: condition diagnosis in any position
E&M visits, direct care, primary/ secondary diagnosis	Number of evaluation and management visits, direct care: target condition diagnosis in any position
Psychotherapy:	
Any psychotherapy, no antidepressants	Flag for any condition-related psychotherapy, no antidepressants
Any evidence-based therapy	Flag for at least one session with evidence-based therapy

Table A.1—continued

Variable	Variable Description
Therapeutic Alliance Questionnaire score	Last DoD/VA Therapeutic Alliance Questionnaire score based on 3-item scale developed by the Army
Group/Individual therapy:	
Group therapy visits, all care, any MH, per month	Number of group therapy sessions, direct care and purchased care PER MONTH: any mental health diagnosis
Group therapy visits, direct care, any MH, per month	Number of group therapy sessions, direct care PER MONTH: any mental health diagnosis
Group therapy visits, all care, primary diagnosis, per month	Number of group therapy sessions, direct care and purchased care PER MONTH: target condition primary diagnosis
Group therapy visits, direct care, primary diagnosis, per month	Number of group therapy sessions, direct care PER MONTH: target condition primary diagnosis
Group therapy visits, all care, primary/secondary diagnosis per month	Number of group therapy sessions, direct care and purchased care PER MONTH: target condition diagnosis in any position
Group therapy visits, direct care, primary/secondary diagnosis, per month	Number of group therapy sessions, direct care PER MONTH: target condition diagnosis in any position
Group therapy visits, all care, primary/secondary diagnosis, per month, categorical	Categorical number of group therapy sessions, direct care and purchased care PER MONTH: target condition diagnosis in any position [0; >0–<3; 3–≤4; >4]
Group therapy visits, direct care, primary/secondary diagnosis, per month, categorical	Categorical number of group therapy sessions, direct care PER MONTH: target condition diagnosis in any position [0; >0–<3; 3–≤4; >4]
Group therapy visits, all care, any MH, per month, categorical	Categorical number of group therapy sessions, direct care and purchased care PER MONTH: any mental health diagnosis [0; >0–<3; 3–≤4; >4]
Group therapy visits, direct care, any MH, per month, categorical	Categorical number of group therapy sessions, direct care PER MONTH: any mental health diagnosis [0; >0–<3; 3–≤4; >4]
Group therapy visits, all care, primary diagnosis, per month, categorical	Categorical number of group therapy sessions, direct care and purchased care PER MONTH: target condition primary diagnosis [0; >0–<3; 3–≤4; >4]
Group therapy visits, direct care, primary diagnosis, per month, categorical	Categorical number of group therapy sessions, direct care PER MONTH: target condition primary diagnosis [0; >0–<3; 3–≤4; >4]
Individual therapy visits, all care, any MH, per month	Number of individual therapy sessions, direct care and purchased care PER MONTH: any mental health diagnosis
Individual therapy visits, direct care, any MH, per month	Number of individual therapy sessions, direct care PER MONTH: any mental health diagnosis

Table A.1—continued

Variable	Variable Description
Individual therapy visits, all care, primary diagnosis, per month	Number of individual therapy sessions, direct care and purchased care PER MONTH: target condition primary diagnosis
Individual therapy visits, direct care, primary diagnosis, per month	Number of individual therapy sessions, direct care PER MONTH: target condition primary diagnosis
Individual therapy visits, all care, primary/secondary diagnosis per month	Number of individual therapy sessions, direct care and purchased care PER MONTH: target condition diagnosis in any position
Individual therapy visits, direct care, primary/secondary diagnosis, per month	Number of individual therapy sessions, direct care PER MONTH: target condition diagnosis in any position
Individual therapy visits, all care, any MH, per month, categorical	Categorical number of individual therapy sessions, direct care and purchased care PER MONTH: any mental health diagnosis [0–<3; 3–4; >4]
Individual therapy visits, direct care, any MH, per month, categorical	Categorical number of individual therapy sessions, direct care PER MONTH: any mental health diagnosis [0–<3; 3–4; >4]
Individual therapy visits, all care, primary/secondary diagnosis, per month, categorical	Categorical number of individual therapy sessions, direct care and purchased care PER MONTH: target condition diagnosis in any position [0–<3; 3–4; >4]
Individual therapy visits, direct care, primary/secondary diagnosis, per month, categorical	Categorical number of individual therapy sessions, direct care PER MONTH: target condition diagnosis in any position [0–<3; 3–4; >4]
Individual therapy visits, all care, primary diagnosis, per month, categorical	Categorical number of individual therapy sessions, direct care and purchased care PER MONTH: target condition primary diagnosis [0–<3; 3–4; >4]
Individual therapy visits, direct care, primary diagnosis, per month, categorical	Categorical number of individual therapy sessions, direct care PER MONTH: target condition primary diagnosis [0–<3; 3–4; >4]

Visits during follow-up period or visits in 90 days:

Variable	Variable Description
Outpatient visits, all care, any MH	Number of outpatient visits, direct care and purchased care: any mental health diagnosis
Outpatient visits, all care, primary diagnosis	Number of outpatient visits, direct care and purchased care: target condition primary diagnosis
Outpatient visits, all care, primary/secondary diagnosis	Number of outpatient visits, direct care and purchased care: target condition diagnosis in any position
Outpatient visits, direct care, any MH	Number of outpatient visits, direct care: any mental health diagnosis

Table A.1—continued

Variable	Variable Description
Outpatient visits, direct care, primary diagnosis	Number of outpatient visits, direct care: target condition primary diagnosis
Outpatient visits, direct care, primary/secondary diagnosis	Number of outpatient visits, direct care: target condition diagnosis in any position
BH visits, direct care, with IOP, any MH per month	Number of outpatient behavioral health visits, direct care (BF clinic, provider type 1 or 2, not TCON), including intensive outpatient program PER MONTH: any mental health diagnosis
BH visits, direct care, with IOP, primary diagnosis per month	Number of outpatient behavioral health visits, direct care (BF clinic, provider type 1 or 2, not TCON), including intensive outpatient program PER MONTH: target condition primary diagnosis
BH visits, direct care, with IOP, primary/secondary diagnosis per month	Number of outpatient behavioral health visits, direct care (BF clinic, provider type 1 or 2, not TCON), including intensive outpatient program PER MONTH: target condition diagnosis in any position
BH visits, direct care, without IOP, any MH per month	Number of outpatient behavioral health visits, direct care (BF clinic, provider type 1 or 2, not TCON), without intensive outpatient program PER MONTH: any mental health diagnosis
BH visits, direct care, without IOP, primary diagnosis per month	Number of outpatient behavioral health visits, direct care (BF clinic, provider type 1 or 2, not TCON), without intensive outpatient program PER MONTH: target condition primary diagnosis
BH visits, direct care, without IOP, primary/secondary diagnosis per month	Number of outpatient behavioral health visits, direct care (BF clinic, provider type 1 or 2, not TCON), without intensive outpatient program PER MONTH: target condition diagnosis in any position
BH visits, direct care, with IOP, any MH, per month, categorical	Categorical number of outpatient behavioral health visits, direct care (BF clinic, provider type 1 or 2, not TCON), including intensive outpatient program PER MONTH: any mental health diagnosis [0–<1.5; 1.5–<2.5; ≥2.5]
BH visits, direct care, with IOP, primary/secondary diagnosis, per month, categorical	Categorical number of outpatient behavioral health visits, direct care (BF clinic, provider type 1 or 2, not TCON), including intensive outpatient program PER MONTH: target condition diagnosis in any position [>0–1.5; 1.5–<2.5; ≥2.5]
BH visits, direct care, without IOP, any MH, per month, categorical	Categorical number of outpatient behavioral health visits, direct care (BF clinic, provider type 1 or 2, not TCON), without intensive outpatient program PER MONTH: any mental health diagnosis [0–<1.5; 1.5–<2.5; ≥2.5]
BH visits, direct care, without IOP, primary/secondary diagnosis, per month, categorical	Categorical number of outpatient behavioral health visits, direct care (BF clinic, provider type 1 or 2, not TCON), without intensive outpatient program PER MONTH: target condition diagnosis in any position [>0–1.5; 1.5–<2.5; ≥2.5]
BH visits, direct care, with IOP, primary diagnosis, per month, categorical	Categorical number of outpatient behavioral health visits, direct care (BF clinic, provider type 1 or 2, not TCON), including intensive outpatient program PER MONTH: target condition primary diagnosis [0–<1.5; 1.5–<2.5; ≥2.5]

Table A.1—continued

Variable	Variable Description
BH visits, direct care, without IOP, primary diagnosis, per month, categorical	Categorical number of outpatient behavioral health visits, direct care (BF clinic, provider type 1 or 2, not TCON), without intensive outpatient program PER MONTH: target condition primary diagnosis [0–<1.5; 1.5–<2.5; ≥2.5]
Visits in 90 days, any MH diagnosis	Number of sessions in 90 days post intake (BF clinic, provider type 1 or 2, not TCON): any mental health diagnosis REGARDLESS of timing of first score
3+ visits, any MH diagnosis	Flag for dosage met: 3+ visits in 90 days after intake (BF clinic, provider type 1 or 2, not TCON): any mental health diagnosis REGARDLESS of timing of first score
Visits in 90 days, primary diagnosis	Number of sessions in 90 days post intake (BF clinic, provider type 1 or 2, not TCON): target condition primary diagnosis REGARDLESS of timing of first score
3+ visits, primary diagnosis	Flag for dosage met: 3+ visits in 90 days after intake (BF clinic, provider type 1 or 2, not TCON): target condition primary diagnosis REGARDLESS of timing of first score
Visits in 90 days, primary/ secondary diagnosis	Number of sessions in 90 days post intake (BF clinic, provider type 1 or 2, not TCON): target condition diagnosis in any position REGARDLESS of timing of first score
3+ visits, primary/secondary diagnosis	Flag for dosage met: 3+ visits in 90 days after intake (BF clinic, provider type 1 or 2, not TCON): target condition diagnosis in any position REGARDLESS of timing of first score
Visits in 90 days, any MH diagnosis, score before intake	Number of sessions in 90 days post intake (BF clinic, provider type 1 or 2, not TCON): any mental health diagnosis ONLY for those with score before intake
3+ visits, any MH diagnosis, score before intake	Flag for dosage met: 3+ visits in 90 days after intake (BF clinic, provider type 1 or 2, not TCON): any mental health diagnosis ONLY for those with score before intake
Visits in 90 days, primary diagnosis, score before intake	Number of sessions in 90 days post intake (BF clinic, provider type 1 or 2, not TCON): target condition primary diagnosis ONLY for those with score before intake
3+ visits, primary diagnosis, score before intake	Flag for dosage met: 3+ visits in 90 days after intake (BF clinic, provider type 1 or 2, not TCON): target condition primary diagnosis ONLY for those with score before intake
Visits in 90 days, primary/ secondary diagnosis, score before intake	Number of sessions in 90 days post intake (BF clinic, provider type 1 or 2, not TCON): target condition diagnosis in any position ONLY for those with score before intake
3+ visits, primary/secondary diagnosis, score before intake	Flag for dosage met: 3+ visits in 90 days after intake (BF clinic, provider type 1 or 2, not TCON): target condition diagnosis in any position ONLY for those with score before intake
3+ visits, any MH diagnosis, type 1 provider	Flag for dosage met: 3+ visits in 90 days after intake (BF clinic, not TCON), any mental health diagnosis: TYPE 1 provider REGARDLESS of timing of first score

Table A.1—continued

Variable	Variable Description
3+ visits, any MH diagnosis, type 2 provider	Flag for dosage met: 3+ visits in 90 days after intake (BF clinic, not TCON), any mental health diagnosis: TYPE 2 provider REGARDLESS of timing of first score
3+ visits, primary diagnosis, type 1 provider	Flag for dosage met: 3+ visits in 90 days after intake (BF clinic, not TCON), target condition primary diagnosis: TYPE 1 provider REGARDLESS of timing of first score
3+ visits, primary diagnosis, type 2 provider	Flag for dosage met: 3+ visits in 90 days after intake (BF clinic, not TCON), target condition primary diagnosis: TYPE 2 provider REGARDLESS of timing of first score
3+ visits, primary/secondary diagnosis, type 1 provider	Flag for dosage met: 3+ visits in 90 days after intake (BF clinic, not TCON), target condition diagnosis in any position TYPE 1 provider REGARDLESS of timing of first score
3+ visits, primary/secondary diagnosis, type 2 provider	Flag for dosage met: 3+ visits in 90 days after intake (BF clinic, not TCON), target condition diagnosis in any position: TYPE 2 provider REGARDLESS of timing of first score
Any MH purchased care	Flag for any purchased care for any mental health diagnosis
Medication:	
Medication for 60 days	Flag for at least 57 days of SSRI/SNRI (for PTSD or anxiety) or antidepressant (for depression) dispensed during any 60 contiguous days from initial score
Any benzodiazepine	Flag for any benzodiazepine dispensed
Benzodiazepine, days' supply, categorical	Categorical benzodiazepine days' supply dispensed [0 days; 1–30 days; >30 days]
Psychotropic drug classes	Number of classes of psychotropic medication dispensed (up to 6): antidepressant, hypnotic/sedative/anxiolytic, antipsychotic, mood stabilizer/anticonvulsant, stimulant, prazosin, other psychotropic
SSRI/SNRI/antidepressant and psychotherapy	Flag for any SSRI/SNRI (PTSD, anxiety) or antidepressant (depression) AND 1 condition-related psychotherapy session after initial score
PTSD	
BH visits, direct care, without IOP, type 1 provider, primary diagnosis per month	Number of outpatient behavioral health visits, direct care (BF clinic, not TCON), provider type 1, without intensive outpatient program PER MONTH: target condition primary diagnosis
BH visits, direct care, without IOP, type 2 provider, primary diagnosis per month	Number of outpatient behavioral health visits, direct care (BF clinic, not TCON), provider type 2, without intensive outpatient program PER MONTH: target condition primary diagnosis
Anxiety	
BH visits, direct care, with IOP, type 1 provider, any MH, per month	Number of outpatient behavioral health visits, direct care (BF clinic, not TCON), provider type 1, including intensive outpatient program PER MONTH: any mental health diagnosis

Table A.1—continued

Variable	Variable Description
BH visits, direct care, with IOP, type 2 provider, any MH, per month	Number of outpatient behavioral health visits, direct care (BF clinic, not TCON), provider type 2, including intensive outpatient program PER MONTH: any mental health diagnosis
Depression	
Individual therapy visits, direct care, type 1 provider, any MH, per month, categorical	Categorical number of individual therapy visits, direct care, provider type 1, PER MONTH: any mental health diagnosis [0–<2; 2–<4; ≥4]
Individual therapy visits, direct care, type 2 provider, any MH, per month, categorical	Categorical number of individual therapy visits, direct care, provider type 2, PER MONTH: any mental health diagnosis [0–<2; 2–<4; ≥4]

PTSD, Depression, and Anxiety Outcome Models: Full Model Results

Table B.1

Pretreatment Predictors of PTSD Symptom Outcomes Among Soldiers in the PTSD Sample (n = 1,759)

Variable	Difference Between First and Last PCL-5 Scores (Continuous)		Response (Dichotomous)		Remission (Dichotomous)	
	Estimate [CI]	P-Value	Odds Ratio [CI]	P-Value	Odds Ratio [CI]	P-Value
Marital status						
Divorced, separated, widowed	1.15 [−2.26, 4.56]	0.51	0.89 [0.56, 1.43]	0.39	0.73 [0.36, 1.47]	0.30
Married	−0.10 [−2.72, 2.52]	0.94	1.11 [0.78, 1.58]	0.25	1.00 [0.61, 1.64]	0.44
Never married [reference group]						
Sex						
Male	1.57 [−0.64, 3.79]	0.16	0.78 [0.58, 1.05]	0.10	0.76 [0.49, 1.18]	0.22
Age						
18–24 [reference group]						
25–34	−0.74 [−3.62, 2.13]	0.61	1.03 [0.70, 1.51]	0.64	0.91 [0.53, 1.55]	0.83
35–44	−0.18 [−3.49, 3.13]	0.92	0.95 [0.61, 1.48]	0.73	0.85 [0.45, 1.62]	0.55
45–64	−1.51 [−5.66, 2.64]	0.47	0.96 [0.55, 1.70]	0.88	0.99 [0.44, 2.24]	0.81
Race/ethnicity						
Black, non-Hispanic	0.52 [−1.31, 2.35]	0.58	0.89 [0.69, 1.15]	0.31	0.93 [0.64, 1.37]	0.54
Hispanic	1.36 [−0.88, 3.60]	0.23	0.79 [0.58, 1.08]	0.07	0.80 [0.50, 1.30]	0.18

Table B.1—continued

Variable	Difference Between First and Last PCL-5 Scores (Continuous)		Response (Dichotomous)		Remission (Dichotomous)	
	Estimate [CI]	P-Value	Odds Ratio [CI]	P-Value	Odds Ratio [CI]	P-Value
Other	−0.29 [−3.40, 2.83]	0.86	1.33 [0.88, 2.02]	0.05	1.46 [0.82, 2.60]	0.10
White, non-Hispanic [reference group]						
Pay grade						
E1–E4	−1.36 [−4.73, 2.01]	0.43	1.11 [0.70, 1.75]	0.29	1.03 [0.53, 2.01]	0.78
E5–E6	1.43 [−1.23, 4.09]	0.29	0.85 [0.59, 1.22]	0.17	0.93 [0.54, 1.61]	0.75
E7–E9	0.77 [−2.12, 3.65]	0.60	0.90 [0.6, 1.33]	0.57	0.93 [0.51, 1.72]	0.82
Officer/warrant officer [reference group]						
Total deployments	0.08 [−0.51, 0.67]	0.79	0.97 [0.89, 1.05]	0.40	0.89 [0.77, 1.02]	0.08
General distress (BASIS score)	5.30 [2.66, 7.94]	0.00	0.49 [0.34, 0.70]	0.00	0.50 [0.30, 0.85]	0.01
Suicide risk (C-SSRS, current score)	−1.05 [−1.74, −0.35]	0.00	1.15 [1.05, 1.26]	0.00	1.08 [0.95, 1.24]	0.25
Alcohol consumption (AUDIT-C score)	−0.33 [−0.60, −0.05]	0.02	1.03 [1.00, 1.07]	0.07	1.08 [1.03, 1.14]	0.00
Function, occupational (WRAIR OF score)	−0.24 [−0.50, 0.03]	0.08	1.05 [1.01, 1.09]	0.01	1.07 [1.02, 1.13]	0.01
Function, personal/social (WRAIR PSF score)	0.43 [0.11, 0.76]	0.01	0.94 [0.90, 0.98]	0.00	0.90 [0.84, 0.96]	0.00
Pain, current	1.22 [−0.53, 2.98]	0.17	0.87 [0.69, 1.10]	0.25	0.82 [0.58, 1.15]	0.24
Initial PCL-5 score	−0.47 [−0.56, −0.38]	0.00	1.04 [1.03, 1.05]	0.00	0.98 [0.96, 1.00]	0.01
PHQ-9 score	−0.26 [−0.51, −0.01]	0.05	1.03 [0.99, 1.06]	0.11	1.01 [0.96, 1.06]	0.66
GAD-7 score	0.11 [−0.14, 0.35]	0.40	1.00 [0.97, 1.04]	0.78	0.98 [0.94, 1.03]	0.53
Anxiety, past history	1.49 [−0.27, 3.26]	0.10	0.87 [0.68, 1.11]	0.26	0.87 [0.60, 1.26]	0.45
Depression, past history	−0.29 [−2.07, 1.49]	0.75	1.01 [0.79, 1.29]	0.95	1.06 [0.73, 1.53]	0.75
PTSD, past history	0.18 [−1.74, 2.09]	0.86	0.98 [0.75, 1.28]	0.87	1.11 [0.74, 1.66]	0.61
Sleep disorder/symptoms, past history	−0.17 [−1.89, 1.55]	0.84	1.00 [0.79, 1.26]	0.98	1.08 [0.76, 1.53]	0.68

Table B.1—continued

Variable	Difference Between First and Last PCL-5 Scores (Continuous)		Response (Dichotomous)		Remission (Dichotomous)	
	Estimate [CI]	P-Value	Odds Ratio [CI]	P-Value	Odds Ratio [CI]	P-Value
Anxiety, current	0.23 [–1.47, 1.92]	0.79	0.95 [0.75, 1.20]	0.66	1.12 [0.79, 1.59]	0.54
Sleep disorder/ symptoms, current	0.93 [–0.68, 2.54]	0.26	0.84 [0.68, 1.05]	0.13	0.79 [0.56, 1.10]	0.16
Psychotropic medication, current[a]	–0.29 [–1.97, 1.39]	0.74	1.00 [0.79, 1.26]	1.00	1.04 [0.74, 1.47]	0.82
Non-MH outpatient visits[b]	0.06 [–0.01, 0.13]	0.08	0.99 [0.98, 1.00]	0.10	0.99 [0.97, 1.01]	0.19
MH outpatient visits[b]	0.04 [0.00, 0.08]	0.07	0.99 [0.99, 1.00]	0.09	0.99 [0.98, 1.00]	0.21

[a] In the 30 days before initial symptom score.

[b] In the 1 year before to 30 days before initial symptom score.

NOTES: Current = 30 days prior to 1 week after initial symptom score; past history = 1 year to 30 days prior to initial symptom score.

Table B.2
Pretreatment Predictors of Depression Symptom Outcomes Among Soldiers in the Depression Sample (n = 1,640)

Variable	Difference Between First and Last PHQ-9 Scores (Continuous)		Response (Dichotomous)		Remission (Dichotomous)	
	Estimate [CI]	P-Value	Odds Ratio [CI]	P-Value	Odds Ratio [CI]	P-Value
Marital status						
Divorced, separated, widowed	1.75 [0.54, 2.95]	0.00	1.19 [0.73, 1.97]	0.38	0.56 [0.31, 0.99]	0.07
Married	1.03 [0.18, 1.88]	0.02	0.98 [0.69, 1.4]	0.47	0.81 [0.57, 1.15]	0.62
Never married [reference group]						
Sex						
Male	0.28 [−0.45, 1.01]	0.45	1.00 [0.74, 1.35]	0.99	0.94 [0.68, 1.31]	0.73
Age						
18–24 [reference group]						
25–34	−0.06 [−1.01, 0.89]	0.90	0.93 [0.63, 1.37]	0.28	1.12 [0.75, 1.68]	0.76
35–44	−0.10 [−1.36, 1.16]	0.87	1.12 [0.67, 1.88]	0.67	1.17 [0.65, 2.09]	0.62
45–64	0.12 [−1.53, 1.76]	0.89	1.19 [0.61, 2.33]	0.56	1.02 [0.46, 2.27]	0.85
Race/ethnicity						
Black, non-Hispanic	0.28 [−0.46, 1.02]	0.46	1.04 [0.76, 1.43]	0.75	0.90 [0.65, 1.25]	0.91
Hispanic	1.15 [0.29, 2.01]	0.01	1.07 [0.75, 1.53]	0.63	0.57 [0.37, 0.88]	0.01
Other	0.02 [−1.19, 1.24]	0.97	0.92 [0.55, 1.53]	0.62	1.20 [0.70, 2.06]	0.14
White, non-Hispanic [reference group]						
Pay grade						
E1–E4	0.10 [−1.23, 1.44]	0.88	1.44 [0.82, 2.54]	0.18	0.76 [0.42, 1.39]	0.58
E5–E6	0.71 [−0.41, 1.83]	0.21	1.12 [0.68, 1.82]	0.77	0.71 [0.42, 1.19]	0.20
E7–E9	0.01 [−1.24, 1.25]	0.99	1.11 [0.64, 1.91]	0.80	0.91 [0.50, 1.65]	0.67
Officer/warrant officer [reference group]						
Total deployments	0.05 [−0.19, 0.30]	0.66	0.94 [0.85, 1.05]	0.28	0.94 [0.83, 1.06]	0.32

Table B.2—continued

Variable	Difference Between First and Last PHQ-9 Scores (Continuous)		Response (Dichotomous)		Remission (Dichotomous)	
	Estimate [CI]	P-Value	Odds Ratio [CI]	P-Value	Odds Ratio [CI]	P-Value
General distress (BASIS score)	0.09 [−0.90, 1.09]	0.86	0.89 [0.58, 1.36]	0.58	1.01 [0.65, 1.55]	0.98
Suicide risk (C-SSRS, current score)	−0.25 [−0.47, −0.03]	0.02	1.00 [0.92, 1.09]	0.98	1.11 [1.01, 1.22]	0.02
Alcohol consumption (AUDIT-C score)	0.04 [−0.07, 0.15]	0.44	1.00 [0.96, 1.05]	0.88	1.00 [0.95, 1.06]	0.93
Function, occupational (WRAIR OF score)	0.04 [−0.06, 0.14]	0.46	0.98 [0.94, 1.02]	0.27	0.99 [0.95, 1.04]	0.80
Function, personal/ social (WRAIR PSF score)	0.23 [0.10, 0.35]	0.00	0.97 [0.92, 1.02]	0.20	0.92 [0.87, 0.97]	0.00
Pain, current	0.98 [0.33, 1.64]	0.00	1.20 [0.91, 1.58]	0.21	0.67 [0.51, 0.89]	0.01
Initial PHQ-9 score	−0.77 [−0.88, −0.67]	0.00	1.30 [1.24, 1.37]	0.00	1.00 [0.96, 1.05]	0.84
GAD-7 score	0.07 [−0.03, 0.16]	0.16	1.00 [0.96, 1.04]	0.83	0.98 [0.94, 1.02]	0.32
PCL-5 score	0.05 [0.02, 0.08]	0.00	0.99 [0.98, 1.01]	0.41	0.99 [0.97, 1.00]	0.03
Anxiety, past history	−0.11 [−0.83, 0.60]	0.76	1.03 [0.76, 1.40]	0.85	0.83 [0.58, 1.19]	0.30
Depression, past history	0.30 [−0.37, 0.96]	0.39	1.13 [0.85, 1.51]	0.40	0.82 [0.59, 1.13]	0.22
PTSD, past history	0.41 [−0.58, 1.41]	0.42	1.11 [0.72, 1.71]	0.62	0.55 [0.31, 0.97]	0.04
Sleep disorder/ symptoms, past history	1.02 [0.33, 1.72]	0.00	1.01 [0.75, 1.36]	0.94	0.56 [0.40, 0.78]	0.00
PTSD, current	0.50 [−0.40, 1.39]	0.27	1.07 [0.73, 1.56]	0.73	0.79 [0.50, 1.26]	0.33
Anxiety, current	0.35 [−0.34, 1.03]	0.32	1.02 [0.76, 1.36]	0.91	0.81 [0.58, 1.12]	0.19
Sleep disorder/ symptoms, current	0.23 [−0.42, 0.88]	0.49	0.91 [0.69, 1.20]	0.51	0.81 [0.60, 1.11]	0.20
Psychotropic medication, current[a]	0.53 [−0.14, 1.21]	0.12	0.99 [0.74, 1.31]	0.92	0.87 [0.64, 1.18]	0.36
Non-MH outpatient visits[b]	0.02 [−0.01, 0.04]	0.21	0.99 [0.98, 1.00]	0.18	0.99 [0.98, 1.01]	0.48
MH outpatient visits[b]	0.01 [−0.01, 0.03]	0.17	0.99 [0.98, 1.00]	0.01	1.00 [0.99, 1.01]	0.64

[a] In the 30 days before initial symptom score.

[b] In the 1 year before to 30 days before initial symptom score.

NOTES: Past history = 1 year to 30 days prior to initial symptom score; current = 30 days prior to 1 week after initial symptom score.

Table B.3
Pretreatment Predictors of Anxiety Symptom Outcomes Among Army Soldiers in the Anxiety Sample (n = 1,828)

Variable	Difference Between First and Last GAD-7 Scores (Continuous)		Response (Dichotomous)		Remission (Dichotomous)	
	Estimate [CI]	P-Value	Odds Ratio [CI]	P-Value	Odds Ratio [CI]	P-Value
Marital status						
Divorced, separated, widowed	1.07 [−0.04, 2.19]	0.06	1.70 [0.92, 3.14]	0.09	0.63 [0.37, 1.04]	0.15
Married	0.81 [0.06, 1.57]	0.04	1.21 [0.77, 1.89]	0.68	0.77 [0.56, 1.04]	0.82
Never married [reference group]						
Sex						
Male	0.10 [−0.57, 0.78]	0.76	0.82 [0.56, 1.2]	0.30	0.80 [0.59, 1.07]	0.13
Age						
18–24 [reference group]						
25–34	0.02 [−0.82, 0.86]	0.97	1.14 [0.72, 1.81]	0.17	0.93 [0.65, 1.32]	0.13
35–44	−0.15 [−1.21, 0.92]	0.79	1.28 [0.70, 2.33]	0.07	0.93 [0.58, 1.48]	0.19
45–64	−0.83 [−2.35, 0.69]	0.29	0.47 [0.16, 1.40]	0.08	1.66 [0.86, 3.19]	0.04
Race/ethnicity						
Black, non-Hispanic	0.84 [0.19, 1.49]	0.01	0.83 [0.57, 1.22]	0.83	0.70 [0.52, 0.94]	0.26
Hispanic	0.53 [−0.24, 1.30]	0.18	0.90 [0.58, 1.41]	0.80	0.92 [0.66, 1.29]	0.28
Other	1.34 [0.27, 2.42]	0.01	0.73 [0.38, 1.43]	0.52	0.63 [0.38, 1.06]	0.22
White, non-Hispanic [reference group]						
Pay grade						
E1–E4	0.32 [−0.85, 1.49]	0.59	1.05 [0.55, 2.00]	0.34	0.92 [0.55, 1.55]	0.50
E5–E6	0.04 [−0.96, 1.03]	0.94	0.72 [0.42, 1.27]	0.16	1.11 [0.71, 1.74]	0.40
E7–E9	0.41 [−0.70, 1.52]	0.47	0.78 [0.41, 1.48]	0.55	1.05 [0.63, 1.75]	0.84
Officer/warrant officer [reference group]						
Total deployments	0.13 [−0.10, 0.35]	0.28	1.05 [0.92, 1.19]	0.45	0.91 [0.82, 1.02]	0.09

Table B.3—continued

Variable	Difference Between First and Last GAD-7 Scores (Continuous)		Response (Dichotomous)		Remission (Dichotomous)	
	Estimate [CI]	P-Value	Odds Ratio [CI]	P-Value	Odds Ratio [CI]	P-Value
General distress (BASIS score)	0.11 [−0.77, 0.99]	0.80	1.04 [0.63, 1.73]	0.87	0.76 [0.52, 1.11]	0.15
Suicide risk (C-SSRS, current score)	−0.14 [−0.39, 0.11]	0.27	1.05 [0.92, 1.20]	0.44	1.08 [0.97, 1.21]	0.16
Alcohol consumption (AUDIT-C score)	−0.05 [−0.15, 0.05]	0.37	1.04 [0.98, 1.10]	0.18	1.02 [0.97, 1.06]	0.48
Function, personal/social (WRAIR PSF score)	0.07 [−0.02, 0.16]	0.14	1.01 [0.96, 1.06]	0.82	0.98 [0.94, 1.02]	0.36
Function, occupational (WRAIR OF score)	0.09 [−0.02, 0.20]	0.12	0.98 [0.92, 1.04]	0.48	0.98 [0.93, 1.03]	0.44
Pain, current	0.79 [0.22, 1.36]	0.01	0.62 [0.45, 0.86]	0.00	0.88 [0.69, 1.12]	0.31
Initial GAD-7 score	−0.66 [−0.76, −0.56]	0.00	1.45 [1.36, 1.54]	0.00	0.97 [0.93, 1.01]	0.19
PHQ-9 score	−0.02 [−0.10, 0.07]	0.68	1.00 [0.95, 1.05]	0.95	1.00 [0.96, 1.03]	0.88
PCL-5 score	0.06 [0.04, 0.09]	0.00	0.98 [0.96, 0.99]	0.00	0.98 [0.97, 1.00]	0.01
PTSD, past history	0.38 [−0.45, 1.20]	0.37	0.90 [0.56, 1.46]	0.68	0.68 [0.45, 1.03]	0.07
Anxiety, past history	0.25 [−0.36, 0.86]	0.43	1.02 [0.71, 1.46]	0.91	0.94 [0.71, 1.25]	0.67
Depression, past history	0.24 [−0.37, 0.86]	0.44	1.04 [0.72, 1.48]	0.85	0.92 [0.70, 1.22]	0.57
PTSD, current	0.29 [−0.46, 1.05]	0.45	1.64 [1.07, 2.50]	0.02	0.69 [0.48, 0.99]	0.04
Sleep disorder/symptoms, past history	0.78 [0.17, 1.39]	0.01	0.95 [0.66, 1.35]	0.76	0.71 [0.54, 0.93]	0.01
Sleep disorder/symptoms, current	0.03 [−0.52, 0.59]	0.91	0.78 [0.56, 1.09]	0.14	1.00 [0.78, 1.28]	0.99
Psychotropic medication, current[a]	0.43 [−0.15, 1.00]	0.14	0.72 [0.51, 1.02]	0.06	0.97 [0.75, 1.25]	0.81
Non-MH outpatient visits[b]	0.01 [−0.01, 0.03]	0.34	1.00 [0.98, 1.01]	0.67	0.99 [0.98, 1.00]	0.14
MH outpatient visits[b]	0.01 [−0.01, 0.03]	0.26	1.00 [0.99, 1.01]	0.46	0.99 [0.99, 1.00]	0.12

[a] In the 30 days before initial symptom score.

[b] In the 1 year before to 30 days before initial symptom score.

NOTES: Past history = 1 year to 30 days prior to initial symptom score; current = 30 days prior to 1 week after initial symptom score.

Table B.4
Pretreatment and Treatment Predictors of PTSD Symptom Outcomes Among Soldiers in the PTSD Sample (n = 1,528)

Variable	Difference Between First and Last PCL-5 Scores (Continuous)		Response (Dichotomous)		Remission (Dichotomous)	
	Estimate [CI]	P-Value	Odds Ratio [CI]	P-Value	Odds Ratio [CI]	P-Value
Time covariates:						
Initial score is after index visit	0.02 [–1.99, 2.03]	0.99	0.82 [0.61, 1.09]	0.18	1.09 [0.73, 1.63]	0.68
Total days between first-last scores	0.05 [0.02, 0.07]	0.00	0.99 [0.99, 1.00]	0.00	1.00 [0.99, 1.00]	0.10
Pretreatment:						
Marital status						
Divorced, separated, widowed	1.59 [–2.10, 5.28]	0.40	0.86 [0.51, 1.44]	0.34	0.52 [0.23, 1.15]	0.09
Married	0.31 [–2.58, 3.20]	0.83	1.11 [0.75, 1.64]	0.24	0.86 [0.50, 1.47]	0.44
Never married [reference group]						
Sex						
Female	–0.61 [–2.94, 1.72]	0.61	1.07 [0.78, 1.47]	0.68	1.02 [0.64, 1.63]	0.94
Age						
18–24	0.52 [–3.88, 4.92]	0.82	1.33 [0.72, 2.44]	0.21	0.95 [0.40, 2.27]	0.90
25–34	1.08 [–2.21, 4.37]	0.52	1.05 [0.66, 1.67]	0.89	0.88 [0.45, 1.72]	0.75
35–44	1.88 [–1.13, 4.89]	0.22	0.92 [0.60, 1.42]	0.20	0.87 [0.47, 1.62]	0.73
45–64 [reference group]						
Race/ethnicity						
Black, non-Hispanic	1.29 [–0.67, 3.25]	0.20	0.87 [0.66, 1.15]	0.35	0.86 [0.57, 1.29]	0.95
Hispanic	2.32 [–0.07, 4.70]	0.06	0.79 [0.56, 1.11]	0.12	0.70 [0.42, 1.17]	0.28
Other	0.96 [–2.27, 4.19]	0.56	1.25 [0.80, 1.94]	0.11	0.93 [0.49, 1.78]	0.75
White, non-Hispanic [reference group]						
Pay grade						
E1–E4	–1.02 [–4.61, 2.57]	0.58	1.15 [0.7, 1.89]	0.55	1.15 [0.55, 2.39]	0.82
E5–E6	0.13 [–2.71, 2.96]	0.93	1.06 [0.71, 1.58]	0.96	1.16 [0.64, 2.13]	0.64
E7–E9	–0.24 [–3.3, 2.83]	0.88	1.00 [0.65, 1.55]	0.73	1.05 [0.54, 2.04]	0.86

Table B.4—continued

Variable	Difference Between First and Last PCL-5 Scores (Continuous)		Response (Dichotomous)		Remission (Dichotomous)	
	Estimate [CI]	P-Value	Odds Ratio [CI]	P-Value	Odds Ratio [CI]	P-Value
Officer/warrant officer [reference group]						
Total deployments	−0.09 [−0.71, 0.53]	0.77	0.99 [0.9, 1.08]	0.75	0.90 [0.78, 1.03]	0.12
General distress (BASIS score)	5.13 [2.46, 7.80]	0.00	0.50 [0.35, 0.73]	0.00	0.55 [0.32, 0.92]	0.02
Suicide risk (C-SSRS, current score)	−1.52 [−2.25, −0.78]	0.00	1.22 [1.10, 1.34]	0.00	1.14 [0.99, 1.32]	0.07
Alcohol consumption (AUDIT-C score)	−0.39 [−0.68, −0.10]	0.01	1.03 [0.99, 1.07]	0.14	1.07 [1.01, 1.14]	0.01
Function, personal/ social (WRAIR PSF score)	0.38 [0.06, 0.69]	0.02	0.95 [0.91, 1.00]	0.04	0.92 [0.86, 0.98]	0.01
Initial PCL-5 score	−0.50 [−0.59, −0.41]	0.00	1.04 [1.03, 1.06]	0.00	0.98 [0.96, 1.00]	0.02
PHQ-9 score	−0.30 [−0.56, −0.04]	0.02	1.04 [1.00, 1.08]	0.05	1.03 [0.98, 1.09]	0.20
Treatment:						
Therapeutic Alliance Questionnaire score	−0.37 [−0.49, −0.25]	0.00	1.03 [1.02, 1.05]	0.00	1.06 [1.03, 1.09]	0.00
Group therapy visits, direct care, primary diagnosis, per month						
>0–<3 visits	3.04 [0.84, 5.24]	0.01	0.60 [0.43, 0.83]	0.03	0.77 [0.47, 1.29]	0.31
3–4 visits	5.56 [−5.63, 16.74]	0.33	0.96 [0.21, 4.36]	0.83	0.65 [0.07, 6.12]	0.51
>4 visits	−5.22 [−14.97, 4.53]	0.29	2.43 [0.66, 8.95]	0.13	3.66 [0.59, 22.67]	0.13
No visits [reference group]						
BH visits, direct care, without IOP, primary diagnosis, per month	1.00 [0.41, 1.58]	0.00	0.93 [0.86, 1.02]	0.11	0.84 [0.74, 0.96]	0.01
Benzodiazepine, days' supply						
0 days [reference group]						
1–30 days	2.09 [−0.69, 4.88]	0.14	0.92 [0.62, 1.36]	0.48	0.84 [0.46, 1.56]	0.63
>30 days	4.24 [1.59, 6.89]	0.00	0.62 [0.42, 0.92]	0.04	0.51 [0.26, 1.01]	0.11
SSRI/SNRI/ antidepressant and psychotherapy	1.84 [0.04, 3.63]	0.04	0.84 [0.66, 1.08]	0.17	0.80 [0.56, 1.14]	0.22

Table B.5
Pretreatment and Treatment Predictors of Depression Symptom Outcomes Among Soldiers in the Depression Sample (n = 1,849)

Variable	Difference Between First and Last PHQ-9 Scores (Continuous)		Response (Dichotomous)		Remission (Dichotomous)	
	Estimate [CI]	P-Value	Odds Ratio [CI]	P-Value	Odds Ratio [CI]	P-Value
Time covariates:						
Initial score is after index visit	0.27 [−0.49, 1.03]	0.49	0.85 [0.60, 1.21]	0.36	0.84 [0.59, 1.18]	0.31
Total days between first-last scores	0.02 [0.02, 0.03]	0.00	1.00 [1.00, 1.00]	0.43	0.99 [0.99, 1.00]	0.00
Pretreatment:						
Marital status						
Divorced, separated, widowed	1.76 [0.63, 2.89]	0.00	0.98 [0.61, 1.60]	0.89	0.54 [0.31, 0.93]	0.08
Married	1.27 [0.47, 2.06]	0.00	0.92 [0.65, 1.29]	0.56	0.70 [0.50, 0.97]	0.73
Never married [reference group]						
Sex						
Female	−0.41 [−1.07, 0.24]	0.21	1.10 [0.84, 1.45]	0.49	1.01 [0.75, 1.37]	0.93
Age						
18–24	0.13 [−1.36, 1.62]	0.86	0.79 [0.42, 1.48]	0.42	0.82 [0.40, 1.67]	0.78
25–34	0.19 [−1.03, 1.40]	0.76	0.92 [0.55, 1.54]	0.89	0.81 [0.45, 1.48]	0.61
35–44	0.25 [−0.89, 1.38]	0.67	0.93 [0.57, 1.51]	0.85	0.83 [0.47, 1.46]	0.81
45–64 [reference group]						
Race/ethnicity						
Black, non-Hispanic	0.24 [−0.43, 0.90]	0.48	1.08 [0.81, 1.45]	0.63	0.85 [0.63, 1.16]	0.89
Hispanic	0.73 [−0.07, 1.52]	0.07	1.15 [0.83, 1.61]	0.36	0.67 [0.46, 0.99]	0.14
Other	0.35 [−0.75, 1.44]	0.54	0.90 [0.55, 1.45]	0.43	0.86 [0.51, 1.44]	0.90
White, non-Hispanic [reference group]						

Table B.5—continued

Variable	Difference Between First and Last PHQ-9 Scores (Continuous)		Response (Dichotomous)		Remission (Dichotomous)	
	Estimate [CI]	P-Value	Odds Ratio [CI]	P-Value	Odds Ratio [CI]	P-Value
Pay grade						
E1–E4	−0.11 [−1.31, 1.09]	0.86	1.54 [0.91, 2.60]	0.15	1.00 [0.58, 1.74]	0.87
E5–E6	0.26 [−0.73, 1.25]	0.61	1.23 [0.79, 1.93]	0.96	0.86 [0.54, 1.38]	0.29
E7–E9	−0.23 [−1.32, 0.86]	0.68	1.24 [0.76, 2.03]	0.99	1.05 [0.62, 1.77]	0.67
Officer/ warrant officer [reference group]						
Total deployments	0.01 [−0.21, 0.24]	0.92	1.03 [0.93, 1.13]	0.58	0.95 [0.85, 1.07]	0.39
Suicide risk (C-SSRS, current score)	−0.37 [−0.56, −0.17]	0.00	1.00 [0.92, 1.09]	0.97	1.20 [1.10, 1.31]	0.00
Function, personal/ social (WRAIR PSF score)	0.23 [0.13, 0.32]	0.00	0.94 [0.91, 0.98]	0.01	0.95 [0.91, 0.99]	0.01
Pain, current	1.01 [0.41, 1.61]	0.00	1.16 [0.89, 1.51]	0.26	0.65 [0.50, 0.85]	0.00
Initial PHQ-9 score	−0.79 [−0.87, −0.71]	0.00	1.27 [1.22, 1.32]	0.00	1.00 [0.96, 1.04]	0.95
PCL-5 score	0.08 [0.06, 0.10]	0.00	0.99 [0.98, 1.00]	0.13	0.98 [0.97, 0.99]	0.00
Sleep disorder/ symptoms, past history	1.33 [0.75, 1.92]	0.00	0.93 [0.72, 1.20]	0.60	0.48 [0.36, 0.65]	0.00
Treatment:						
Therapeutic Alliance Questionnaire score	−0.19 [−0.23, −0.15]	0.00	1.02 [1.01, 1.04]	0.01	1.07 [1.04, 1.09]	0.00
Individual therapy visits, all care, any MH, per month						
0–<2 visits	−1.52 [−2.46, −0.57]	0.00	0.86 [0.57, 1.27]	0.51	2.29 [1.39, 3.77]	0.00
2–4 visits	−0.98 [−1.89, −0.07]	0.03	0.88 [0.60, 1.29]	0.71	1.61 [0.99, 2.60]	0.70
>4 visits [reference group]						

Table B.5—continued

Variable	Difference Between First and Last PHQ-9 Scores (Continuous)		Response (Dichotomous)		Remission (Dichotomous)	
	Estimate [CI]	P-Value	Odds Ratio [CI]	P-Value	Odds Ratio [CI]	P-Value
BH visits, direct care, with IOP, primary/secondary diagnosis, per month	0.10 [−0.07, 0.28]	0.25	0.90 [0.82, 0.98]	0.02	1.03 [0.95, 1.13]	0.48
BH visits, direct care, without IOP, primary diagnosis, per month	−0.14 [−0.41, 0.13]	0.31	1.12 [0.99, 1.27]	0.08	1.01 [0.89, 1.14]	0.92
Benzodiazepine, days' supply						
0 days [reference group]						
1–30 days	0.96 [−0.11, 2.02]	0.08	0.71 [0.45, 1.13]	0.35	1.05 [0.61, 1.80]	0.69
>30 days	0.96 [0.04, 1.88]	0.04	0.81 [0.54, 1.22]	0.85	0.87 [0.53, 1.42]	0.55

NOTE: Past history = 1 year to 30 days prior to initial symptom score; current = 30 days prior to 1 week after initial symptom score.

Table B.6
Pretreatment and Treatment Predictors of Anxiety Symptom Outcomes Among Soldiers in the Anxiety Sample (n = 2,592)

Variable	Difference Between First and Last GAD-7 Scores (Continuous)		Response (Dichotomous)		Remission (Dichotomous)	
	Estimate [CI]	P-Value	Odds Ratio [CI]	P-Value	Odds Ratio [CI]	P-Value
Time covariates:						
Initial score is after index visit	0.02 [−0.56, 0.59]	0.95	1.03 [0.72, 1.45]	0.89	1.00 [0.78, 1.29]	1.00
Total days between first-last scores	0.01 [0.00, 0.01]	0.04	1.00 [1.00, 1.00]	0.26	1.00 [1.00, 1.00]	0.75
Pretreatment:						
Marital status						
Divorced, separated, widowed	1.17 [0.24, 2.11]	0.01	0.92 [0.53, 1.58]	0.46	0.79 [0.52, 1.20]	0.44
Married	0.64 [−0.01, 1.28]	0.05	1.19 [0.83, 1.72]	0.15	0.83 [0.63, 1.08]	0.55
Never married [reference group]						
Sex						
Female	0.01 [−0.53, 0.54]	0.98	1.42 [1.06, 1.90]	0.02	0.99 [0.78, 1.25]	0.91
Age						
18–24	0.36 [−0.85, 1.56]	0.56	1.06 [0.52, 2.18]	0.71	1.00 [0.59, 1.70]	0.47
25–34	0.45 [−0.56, 1.46]	0.38	1.21 [0.64, 2.26]	0.59	0.91 [0.58, 1.44]	0.94
35–44	0.65 [−0.30, 1.61]	0.18	1.29 [0.70, 2.37]	0.34	0.74 [0.48, 1.14]	0.05
45–64 [reference group]						
Race/ethnicity						
Black, non-Hispanic	0.92 [0.39, 1.45]	0.00	0.89 [0.65, 1.21]	0.50	0.65 [0.51, 0.83]	0.14
Hispanic	0.76 [0.12, 1.40]	0.02	1.10 [0.78, 1.57]	0.30	0.79 [0.59, 1.05]	0.71
Other	1.06 [0.16, 1.95]	0.02	0.87 [0.52, 1.45]	0.60	0.63 [0.41, 0.98]	0.28

Table B.6—continued

Variable	Difference Between First and Last GAD-7 Scores (Continuous)		Response (Dichotomous)		Remission (Dichotomous)	
	Estimate [CI]	P-Value	Odds Ratio [CI]	P-Value	Odds Ratio [CI]	P-Value
White, non-Hispanic [reference group]						
Pay grade						
E1–E4	0.39 [–0.55, 1.33]	0.42	0.97 [0.58, 1.62]	0.70	0.90 [0.59, 1.37]	0.65
E5–E6	0.46 [–0.32, 1.24]	0.25	0.77 [0.50, 1.20]	0.12	0.86 [0.61, 1.22]	0.24
E7–E9	0.17 [–0.69, 1.03]	0.70	0.93 [0.57, 1.51]	0.90	1.06 [0.72, 1.56]	0.37
Officer/ warrant officer [reference group]						
Total deployments	0.13 [–0.05, 0.31]	0.17	1.02 [0.92, 1.14]	0.72	0.96 [0.89, 1.04]	0.35
Pain, current	0.95 [0.49, 1.41]	0.00	0.71 [0.55, 0.93]	0.01	0.78 [0.64, 0.95]	0.01
Initial GAD-7 score	–0.69 [–0.76, –0.61]	0.00	1.40 [1.33, 1.47]	0.00	0.99 [0.96, 1.03]	0.67
PCL-5 score	0.08 [0.06, 0.09]	0.00	0.99 [0.98, 1.00]	0.02	0.97 [0.97, 0.98]	0.00
Sleep disorder/ symptoms, past history	0.97 [0.52, 1.43]	0.00	0.93 [0.71, 1.20]	0.57	0.68 [0.55, 0.84]	0.00
Treatment:						
Therapeutic Alliance Questionnaire score	–0.11 [–0.14, –0.08]	0.00	1.01 [0.99, 1.03]	0.17	1.05 [1.04, 1.07]	0.00
Individual therapy visits, direct care, primary/secondary diagnosis, per month	0.06 [–0.19, 0.32]	0.63	1.12 [0.97, 1.29]	0.12	0.99 [0.88, 1.12]	0.93
BH visits, direct care, with IOP, any MH, per month	0.16 [0.08, 0.25]	0.00	1.02 [0.97, 1.07]	0.45	0.90 [0.86, 0.95]	0.00
Any MH purchased care	0.60 [–0.02, 1.21]	0.06	0.72 [0.50, 1.03]	0.07	0.92 [0.69, 1.24]	0.59

Table B.6—continued

Variable	Difference Between First and Last GAD-7 Scores (Continuous)		Response (Dichotomous)		Remission (Dichotomous)	
	Estimate [CI]	P-Value	Odds Ratio [CI]	P-Value	Odds Ratio [CI]	P-Value
Benzodiazepine, days' supply						
0 days [reference group]						
1–30 days	0.21 [−0.56, 0.97]	0.60	0.95 [0.62, 1.45]	0.61	0.87 [0.61, 1.24]	0.87
>30 days	0.76 [0.08, 1.44]	0.03	1.12 [0.78, 1.62]	0.47	0.81 [0.59, 1.11]	0.41

NOTE: Past history = 1 year to 30 days prior to initial symptom score.

References

American Psychiatric Association, "Practice Guidelines for the Treatment of Patients with Panic Disorder," Washington, D.C., 2009.

American Psychiatric Association, "Practice Guideline for the Treatment of Patients with Major Depressive Disorder, Third Edition," 2015. As of October 15, 2018:
https://www.guidelinecentral.com/summaries/
practice-guideline-for-the-treatment-of-patients-with-major-depressive-disorder-third-edition/

Angstman, Kurt B., James E. Rohrer, and Norman H. Rasmussen, "PHQ-9 Response Curve: Rate of Improvement for Depression Treatment with Collaborative Care Management," *Journal of Primary Care & Community Health*, Vol. 3, No. 3, 2012, pp. 155–158.

Army Medicine Public Affairs, "Behavioral Health Data Portal IT Team Winners of the Excellence in Enterprise Information Award," 2013. As of January 25, 2018:
https://www.army.mil/article/113541/
behavioral_health_data_portal_it_team_winners_of_the_excellence_in_enterprise_information_
award

Bandelow, Borwin, Sophie Michaelis, and Dirk Wedekind, "Treatment of Anxiety Disorders," *Dialogues in Clinical Neuroscience*, Vol. 19, No. 2, June 2017, pp. 93–107.

Bandelow, Borwin, Joseph Zohar, Eric Hollander, Siegfried Kasper, Hans-Jürgen Möller, and WFSBP Task Force on Treatment Guidelines for Anxiety Obsessive-Compulsive Post-Traumatic Stress Disorders, "World Federation of Societies of Biological Psychiatry (WFSBP) Guidelines for the Pharmacological Treatment of Anxiety, Obsessive-Compulsive and Post-Traumatic Stress Disorders–First Revision," *The World Journal of Biological Psychiatry*, Vol. 9, No. 4, 2008, pp. 248–312.

Blevins, Christy A., Frank W. Weathers, Margaret T. Davis, Tracy K. Witte, and Jessica L. Domino, "The Posttraumatic Stress Disorder Checklist for DSM-5 (PCL-5): Development and Initial Psychometric Evaluation," *Journal of Traumatic Stress*, Vol. 28, No. 6, December 2015, pp. 489–498.

Boswell, James F., David R. Kraus, Scott D. Miller, and Michael J. Lambert, "Implementing Routine Outcome Monitoring in Clinical Practice: Benefits, Challenges, and Solutions," *Psychotherapy Research*, Vol. 25, No. 1, 2015, pp. 6–19.

Bovin, Michelle J., Brian P. Marx, Frank W. Weathers, Matthew W. Gallagher, Paola Rodriguez, Paula P. Schnurr, and Terence M. Keane, "Psychometric Properties of the PTSD Checklist for Diagnostic and Statistical Manual of Mental Disorders–Fifth Edition (PCL-5) in Veterans," *Psychological Assessment*, Vol. 28, No. 11, November 2016, pp. 1379–1391.

Bush, Kristen, Daniel R. Kivlahan, Mary B. McDonell, Stephan D. Fihn, and Katharine A. Bradley, "The AUDIT Alcohol Consumption Questions (AUDIT-C): An Effective Brief Screening Test for Problem Drinking," *Archives of Internal Medicine*, Vol. 158, No. 16, September 14, 1998, pp. 1789–1795.

Cornum, Rhonda, Michael D. Matthews, and Martin E. P. Seligman, "Comprehensive Soldier Fitness," *Master Resilience Trainer Course Conference*, Philadelphia, Pa., 2009, pp. 7–17.

Cuijpers, Pim, Marcus Huibers, David Daniel Ebert, Sander L. Koole, and Gerhard Andersson, "How Much Psychotherapy Is Needed to Treat Depression? A Metaregression Analysis," *Journal of Affective Disorders*, Vol. 149, No. 1–3, 2013, pp. 1–13.

DoD—*See* U.S. Department of Defense.

DoD, VA, and DHHS—*See* U.S. Department of Defense, U.S. Department of Veterans Affairs, and U.S. Department of Health and Human Services.

Draper, Norman R., and Harry Smith, *Applied Regression Analysis*, 2nd ed., New York: John Wiley & Sons, 1981.

Dursa, Erin K., Matthew J. Reinhard, Shannon K. Barth, and Aaron I. Schneiderman, "Prevalence of a Positive Screen for PTSD Among OEF/OIF and OEF/OIF-Era Veterans in a Large Population-Based Cohort," *Journal of Traumatic Stress*, Vol. 27, No. 5, 2014, pp. 542–549.

Eisen, Susan V., Sharon-Lise Normand, Albert J. Belanger, Avron Spiro, and David Esch, "The Revised Behavior and Symptom Identification Scale (BASIS-R): Reliability and Validity," *Medical Care*, Vol. 42, No. 12, 2004, pp. 1230–1241.

Erickson, Julie, D. Jolene Kinley, Tracie O. Afifi, Mark A. Zamorski, Robert H. Pietrzak, Murray B. Stein, and Jitender Sareen, "Epidemiology of Generalized Anxiety Disorder in Canadian Military Personnel," *Journal of Military, Veteran and Family Health*, Vol. 1, No. 1, 2015, pp. 26–36.

Elvins, Rachel, and Jonathan Green, "The Conceptualization and Measurement of Therapeutic Alliance: An Empirical Review," *Clinical Psychology Review*, Vol. 28, No. 7, 2008, pp. 1167–1187.

Ferreira, Paulo H., Manuela L. Ferreira, Christopher G. Maher, Kathryn M. Refshauge, Jane Latimer, and Roger D. Adams, "The Therapeutic Alliance Between Clinicians and Patients Predicts Outcome in Chronic Low Back Pain," *Physical Therapy*, Vol. 93, No. 4, 2013, pp. 470–478.

Fortney, John C., Jürgen Unützer, Glenda Wrenn, Jeffrey M. Pyne, G. Richard Smith, Michael Schoenbaum, and Henry T. Harbin, "A Tipping Point for Measurement-Based Care," *Psychiatric Services*, Vol. 68, No. 2, 2016, pp. 179–188.

Flückiger, Christoph, A. C. Del Re, Bruce E. Wampold, and Adam O. Horvath, "The Alliance in Adult Psychotherapy: A Meta-Analytic Synthesis," *Psychotherapy*, Vol. 55, No. 4, 2018, pp. 316–340.

Gadermann, Anne M., Charles C. Engel, James A. Naifeh, Matthew K. Nock, Maria Petukhova, Patcho N. Santiago, Benjamin Wu, Alan M. Zaslavsky, and Ronald C. Kessler, "Prevalence of DSM-IV Major Depression Among U.S. Military Personnel: Meta-Analysis and Simulation," *Military Medicine*, Vol. 177, No. 8, 2012, pp. 47–59.

Gartlehner, Gerald, Gernot Wagner, Nina Matyas, Viktoria Titscher, Judith Greimel, Linda Lux, Bradley N. Gaynes, Meera Viswanathan, Sheila Patel, and Kathleen N. Lohr, "Pharmacological and Non-Pharmacological Treatments for Major Depressive Disorder: Review of Systematic Reviews," *BMJ Open*, Vol. 7, No. 6, 2017, p. e014912.

Goodman, Leo A., "Exploratory Latent Structure Analysis Using Both Identifiable and Unidentifiable Models," *Biometrika*, Vol. 61, No. 2, 1974, pp. 215–231.

Guina, Jeffrey, Sarah R. Rossetter, Bethany J. DeRhodes, Ramzi W. Nahhas, and Randon S. Welton, "Benzodiazepines for PTSD: A Systematic Review and Meta-Analysis," *Journal of Psychiatric Practice*, Vol. 21, No. 4, 2015, pp. 281–303.

Haagen, Joris F. G., Geert E. Smid, Jeroen W. Knipscheer, and Rolf J. Kleber, "The Efficacy of Recommended Treatments for Veterans with PTSD: A Metaregression Analysis," *Clinical Psychology Review*, Vol. 40, 2015, pp. 184–194.

Hagenaars, Jacques A., and Allan L. McCutcheon, *Applied Latent Class Analysis*, New York: Cambridge University Press, 2002.

Hall, Amanda M., Paulo H. Ferreira, Christopher G. Maher, Jane Latimer, and Manuela L. Ferreira, "The Influence of the Therapist-Patient Relationship on Treatment Outcome in Physical Rehabilitation: A Systematic Review," *Physical Therapy*, Vol. 90, No. 8, 2010, pp. 1099–1110.

Hatcher, Robert L., and J. Arthur Gillaspy, "Development and Validation of a Revised Short Version of the Working Alliance Inventory," *Psychotherapy Research*, Vol. 16, No. 1, 2006, pp. 12–25.

Headquarters, U.S. Department of the Army, Office of the Surgeon General/U.S. Army Medical Command Policy Memo 14-094, "Policy Guidance on the Assessment and Treatment of PTSD," December 18, 2014.

Hepner, Kimberly A., Coreen Farris, Carrie M. Farmer, Praise O. Iyiewuare, Terri Tanielian, Asa Wilks, Michael Robbins, Susan M. Paddock, and Harold Alan Pincus, *Delivering Clinical Practice Guideline–Concordant Care for PTSD and Major Depression in Military Treatment Facilities*, Santa Monica, Calif.: RAND Corporation, RR-1692-OSD, 2017. As of May 23, 2018:
https://www.rand.org/pubs/research_reports/RR1692.html

Hepner, Kimberly A., Carol P. Roth, Elizabeth M. Sloss, Susan M. Paddock, Praise O. Iyiewuare, Martha J. Timmer, and Harold Alan Pincus, *Quality of Care for PTSD and Depression in the Military Health System: Final Report*, Santa Monica, Calif.: RAND Corporation, RR-1542-OSD, 2017. As of February 18, 2016:
https://www.rand.org/pubs/research_reports/RR1542.html

Hepner, Kimberly A., Elizabeth M. Sloss, Carol P. Roth, Heather Krull, Susan M. Paddock, Shaela Moen, Martha J. Timmer, and Harold Alan Pincus, *Quality of Care for PTSD and Depression in the Military Health System: Phase 1 Report*, Santa Monica, Calif.: RAND Corporation, RR-978-OSD, 2016. As of February 18, 2016:
http://www.rand.org/pubs/research_reports/RR978.html

Hocking, Ronald R., "The Analysis and Selection of Variables in Linear Regression," *Biometrics*, Vol. 32, No. 1, 1976, pp. 1–49.

Hofmann, Stefan G., Anu Asnaani, Imke J. J. Vonk, Alice T. Sawyer, and Angela Fang, "The Efficacy of Cognitive Behavioral Therapy: A Review of Meta-Analyses," *Cognitive Therapy and Research*, Vol. 36, No. 5, 2012, pp. 427–440.

Hoge, Charles W., Christopher G. Ivany, Edward A. Brusher, Millard D. Brown III, John C. Shero, Amy B. Adler, Christopher H. Warner, and David T. Orman, "Transformation of Mental Health Care for U.S. Soldiers and Families During the Iraq and Afghanistan Wars: Where Science and Politics Intersect," *American Journal of Psychiatry*, Vol. 173, No. 4, November 2015, pp. 334–343.

Horvath, Adam O., A. C. Del Re, Christoph Flückiger, and Dianne Symonds, "Alliance in Individual Psychotherapy," *Psychotherapy*, Vol. 48, No. 1, March 2011, pp. 9–16.

Institute of Medicine, *Treatment for Posttraumatic Stress Disorder in Military and Veteran Populations: Final Assessment*, Washington, D.C.: National Academies Press, 2014.

International Consortium for Health Outcomes Measurement (ICHOM), *Depression & Anxiety Data Collection Reference Guide*, Cambridge, Mass.: International Consortium for Health Outcomes Measurement, 2015. As of November 5, 2018:
http://www.ichom.org/medical-conditions/depression-anxiety/

Jensen-Doss, Amanda, Emily M. Becker Haimes, Ashley M. Smith, Aaron R. Lyon, Cara C. Lewis, Cameo F. Stanick, and Kristin M. Hawley, "Monitoring Treatment Progress and Providing Feedback Is Viewed Favorably but Rarely Used in Practice," *Administration and Policy in Mental Health and Mental Health Services Research*, Vol. 45, No. 1, 2018, pp. 48–61.

Keefe, John R., Kevin S. McCarthy, Ulrike Dinger, Sigal Zilcha-Mano, and Jacques P. Barber, "A Meta-Analytic Review of Psychodynamic Therapies for Anxiety Disorders," *Clinical Psychology Review*, Vol. 34, No. 4, 2014, pp. 309–323.

Kelley, John M., Gordon Kraft-Todd, Lidia Schapira, Joe Kossowsky, and Helen Riess, "The Influence of the Patient-Clinician Relationship on Healthcare Outcomes: A Systematic Review and Meta-Analysis of Randomized Controlled Trials," *PLOS One*, Vol. 9, No. 4, 2014, p. e94207.

The Kennedy Forum, *A Core Set of Outcome Measures for Behavioral Health Across Service Settings: Supplement to Fixing Behavioral Health Care in America: A National Call for Measurement-Based Care in the Delivery of Behavioral Health Services*, Chicago: The Kennedy Forum, 2015. As of November 5, 2018:
http://thekennedyforum-dot-org.s3.amazonaws.com/documents/MBC_supplement.pdf

Kroenke, Kurt, Robert L. Spitzer, and Janet B. W. Williams, "The PHQ-9: Validity of a Brief Depression Severity Measure," *Journal of General Internal Medicine*, Vol. 16, No. 9, 2001, pp. 606–613.

Kroll, David S., Harry Reyes Nieva, Arthur J. Barsky, and Jeffrey A. Linder, "Benzodiazepines Are Prescribed More Frequently to Patients Already at Risk for Benzodiazepine-Related Adverse Events in Primary Care," *Journal of General Internal Medicine*, Vol. 31, No. 9, 2016, pp. 1027–1034.

Lo, Yungtai, Nancy R. Mendell, and Donald B. Rubin, "Testing the Number of Components in a Normal Mixture," *Biometrika*, Vol. 88, No. 3, October 2001, pp. 767–778.

Löwe, Bernd, Jürgen Unützer, Christopher M. Callahan, Anthony J. Perkins, and Kurt Kroenke, "Monitoring Depression Treatment Outcomes with the Patient Health Questionnaire-9," *Medical Care*, Vol. 42, No. 12, December 2004, pp. 1194–1201.

Martin, Daniel J., John P. Garske, and M. Katherine Davis, "Relation of the Therapeutic Alliance with Outcome and Other Variables: A Meta-Analytic Review," *Journal of Consulting and Clinical Psychology*, Vol. 68, No. 3, June 2000, pp. 438–450.

Milanak, Melissa E., Daniel F. Gros, Kathryn M. Magruder, Olga Brawman-Mintzer, and B. Christopher Frueh, "Prevalence and Features of Generalized Anxiety Disorder in Department of Veteran Affairs Primary Care Settings," *Psychiatry Research*, Vol. 209, No. 2, 2013, pp. 173–179.

Military Health System Communications Office, "Military Providers Seek Tailored Approach to Treating PTSD," 2018. As of October 15, 2018:
https://health.mil/News/Articles/2018/03/14/
Military-providers-seek-tailored-approach-to-treating-PTSD

MN Community Measurement, *2016 Health Care Quality Report: Compare Clinic, Medical Group and Hospital Performance*, Minneapolis, Minn., 2016. As of September 11, 2018:
http://mncm.org/wp-content/uploads/2017/03/
2016-Health-Care-Quality-Report-Final-3.1.2017-part-1.pdf

MN Community Measurement, "Health Care Quality Report," 2017. As of September 11, 2018:
http://mncm.org/reports-and-websites/reports-and-data/health-care-quality-report/

National Committee for Quality Assurance, "HEDIS Measures and Technical Resources," 2018. As of September 11, 2018:
http://www.ncqa.org/hedis-quality-measurement/hedis-measures/hedis-2017

National Quality Forum, "Quality Positioning System," 2018. As of September 11, 2018: https://www.qualityforum.org/QPS/

Norman, Sonya B., Susan R. Tate, Kendall C. Wilkins, Kevin Cummins, and Sandra A. Brown, "Posttraumatic Stress Disorder's Role in Integrated Substance Dependence and Depression Treatment Outcomes," *Journal of Substance Abuse Treatment*, Vol. 38, No. 4, 2010, pp. 346–355.

NQF—*See* National Quality Forum.

Nylund, Karen L., Tihomir Asparouhov, and Bengt O. Muthén, "Deciding on the Number of Classes in Latent Class Analysis and Growth Mixture Modeling: A Monte Carlo Simulation Study," *Structural Equation Modeling*, Vol. 14, No. 4, 2007, pp. 535–569.

Pietrzak, Eva, Stephen Pullman, Cristina Cotea, and Peter Nasveld, "Effects of Deployment on Mental Health in Modern Military Forces: A Review of Longitudinal Studies," *Journal of Military and Veterans Health*, Vol. 20, No. 3, 2012, pp. 24–36.

Raftery, Adrian E., "Bayesian Model Selection in Structural Equation Models," in Ken Bollen and J. Scott Long, eds., *Testing Structural Equation Models*, Newbury Park, Calif.: Sage Publications, 1993, pp. 163–180.

Seal, Karen H., Thomas J. Metzler, Kristian S. Gima, Daniel Bertenthal, Shira Maguen, and Charles R. Marmar, "Trends and Risk Factors for Mental Health Diagnoses Among Iraq and Afghanistan Veterans Using Department of Veterans Affairs Health Care, 2002–2008," *American Journal of Public Health*, Vol. 99, No. 9, 2009, pp. 1651–1658.

Spitzer, Robert L., Kurt Kroenke, Janet B. W. Williams, and Bernd Löwe, "A Brief Measure for Assessing Generalized Anxiety Disorder: The GAD-7," *Archives of Internal Medicine*, Vol. 166, No. 10, 2006, pp. 1092–1097.

Spitzer, Robert L., Kurt Kroenke, Janet B. W. Williams, and Patient Health Questionnaire Primary Care Study Group, "Validation and Utility of a Self-Report Version of PRIME-MD: The PHQ Primary Care Study," *Journal of the American Medical Association*, Vol. 282, No. 18, November 10, 1999, pp. 1737–1744.

Steenkamp, Maria M., Brett T. Litz, Charles W. Hoge, and Charles R. Marmar, "Psychotherapy for Military-Related PTSD: A Review of Randomized Clinical Trials," *JAMA*, Vol. 314, No. 5, 2015, pp. 489–500.

Sullivan, Patrick F., Michael C. Neale, and Kenneth S. Kendler, "Genetic Epidemiology of Major Depression: Review and Meta-Analysis," *American Journal of Psychiatry*, Vol. 157, No. 10, 2000, pp. 1552–1562.

U.S. Army Medical Command, *Fragmentary Order 3 to Operations Order 12-47 (Behavioral Health Data Portal (BHDP) Implementation)*, Washington, D.C., 2015.

U.S. Department of Defense, *Report to Armed Services Committees of the Senate and House of Representatives; Section 729 of the National Defense Authorization Act for Fiscal Year 2016 (Public Law 114-92): Plan for Development of Procedures to Measure Data on Mental Health Care Provided by the Department of Defense*, Washington, D.C., 2016. As of May 18, 2018: https://health.mil/Reference-Center/Reports/2016/09/13/Plan-for-Development-of-Procedures-to-Measure

U.S. Department of Defense, Deployment Health Clinical Center, *Mental Health Disorder Prevalence Among Active Duty Service Members in the Military Health System, Fiscal Years 2005–2016*, January 2017. As of January 17, 2018: http://www.pdhealth.mil/sites/default/files/images/mental-health-disorder-prevalence-among-active-duty-service-members-508.pdf

U.S. Department of Defense, U.S. Department of Veterans Affairs, and U.S. Department of Health and Human Services, *Interagency Task Force on Military and Veterans Mental Health, 2016 Annual Report*, Washington, D.C., 2016. As of January 23, 2018:
https://www.mentalhealth.va.gov/docs/ITF_2016_Annual_Report_November_2016.pdf

U.S. Department of Veterans Affairs and U.S. Department of Defense, "VA/DoD Clinical Practice Guideline for the Management of Major Depressive Disorder, Version 3.0-2016," 2016. As of January 26, 2018:
https://www.healthquality.va.gov/guidelines/MH/mdd/VADoDMDDCPGFINAL82916.pdf

U.S. Department of Veterans Affairs and U.S. Department of Defense, "VA/DoD Clinical Practice Guideline for Management of PostTraumatic Stress Disorder and Acute Stress Disorder, Version 3.0-2017," 2017. As of October 10, 2018:
https://www.healthquality.va.gov/guidelines/MH/ptsd/VADoDPTSDCPGFinal012418.pdf

VA and DoD—*See* U.S. Department of Veterans Affairs and U.S. Department of Defense.

Valenstein, Marcia, Kiran Khanujua Taylor, Karen Austin, Helen C. Kales, John F. McCarthy, and Frederic C. Blow, "Benzodiazepine Use Among Depressed Patients Treated in Mental Health Settings," *American Journal of Psychiatry*, Vol. 161, No. 4, 2004, pp. 654–661.

van Minnen, Agnes, Lori A. Zoellner, Melanie S. Harned, and Katherine Mills, "Changes in Comorbid Conditions After Prolonged Exposure for PTSD: A Literature Review," *Current Psychiatry Reports*, Vol. 17, No. 3, 2015, p. 549.

Weathers, F. W., B. T. Litz, T. M. Keane, P. A. Palmieri, B. P. Marx, and P. P. Schnurr, "The PTSD Checklist for DSM-5 (PCL-5)," 2013. As of October 10, 2018:
https://www.ptsd.va.gov/professional/assessment/adult-sr/ptsd-checklist.asp

Woodson, Jonathan, Assistant Secretary of Defense for Health Affairs, "Military Treatment Facility Mental Health Clinical Outcomes Guidance," memorandum, September 9, 2013.

Woolaway-Bickel, Kelly, email discussion with Kimberly Hepner on Army's Behavioral Health Service Line tracking of benzodiazepines and atypical antipsychotic prescriptions for PTSD, March 13, 2019.

Xue, Chen, Yang Ge, Bihan Tang, Yuan Liu, Peng Kang, Meng Wang, and Lulu Zhang, "A Meta-Analysis of Risk Factors for Combat-Related PTSD Among Military Personnel and Veterans," *PLOS One*, Vol. 10, No. 3, 2015, p. e0120270.